I0084463

# Fundamentals of the
# Psychiatric Mental Status
# Examination

# Fundamentals of the Psychiatric Mental Status Examination

## A WORKBOOK

Cheryl Webster Pollard

**CANADIAN SCHOLARS**

Toronto | Vancouver

**Fundamentals of the Psychiatric Mental Status Examination: A Workbook**
Cheryl Webster Pollard

First published in 2018 by
**Canadian Scholars, an imprint of CSP Books Inc.**
425 Adelaide Street West, Suite 200
Toronto, Ontario
M5V 3C1

**www.canadianscholars.ca**

Copyright © 2018 Cheryl Webster Pollard and Canadian Scholars.

All rights reserved. No part of this publication may be reproduced, stored in a retrieval system, or transmitted, in any form or by any means, without the prior written permission of Canadian Scholars, under licence or terms from the appropriate reproduction rights organization, or as expressly permitted by law.

Every reasonable effort has been made to identify copyright holders. Canadian Scholars would be pleased to have any errors or omissions brought to its attention.

**Library and Archives Canada Cataloguing in Publication**

Pollard, Cheryl L., author
        Fundamentals of the psychiatric mental status examination : a workbook
/ Cheryl Webster Pollard.

Issued in print and electronic formats.
ISBN 978-1-77338-070-4 (softcover).--ISBN 978-1-77338-071-1 (PDF).--
ISBN 978-1-77338-072-8 (EPUB)

        1. Mental status examination--Problems, exercises, etc.  2. Interviewing in psychiatry--Problems, exercises, etc.  3. Psychodiagnostics--Problems, exercises, etc.  I. Title.

RC469.P65 2018                    616.89'075                    C2018-903659-1
                                                                 C2018-903660-5

Text and cover design by Elisabeth Springate


18   19   20   21   22          5   4   3   2   1


Canada

# Contents

# Acknowledgements

I am truly grateful for the wondrous generosity of my colleagues. You all graciously shared your expertise and time by providing me with feedback on my ideas and helped to clarify my thinking. Although many people provided me with encouragement, I do need to identify some specific individuals who kept reminding me of my task and providing me with guidance. A debt of gratitude goes to Linda Cavanaugh, who charitably shared her teaching expertise and ensured that I stayed focused on providing information that would be useful, and practical, for a beginning or novice clinician. I also need to acknowledge Natalie Garriga, from Canadian Scholars, for her unending patience. Finally, to my family, thank you for giving me space and time to write—it is deeply appreciated.

# Preface

The psychiatric mental status examination is an important assessment. It is used to assess people who may be experiencing changes in their mental well-being. These changes may include, but are not limited to, feelings of sadness, anxiety, worry, or fear. The mental status examination is most commonly used in the fields of mental health and psychiatry; however, as it is a structured assessment that can be used to gather relevant clinical information regardless of the health care setting, it is a valuable tool for all professionals. Although the examples used in this book draw heavily on mental health and psychiatry, the mental status examination is also used regularly by health care professionals working in the areas of emergency medicine, surgery, home care, rehabilitation, public health, and long-term care.

A psychiatric mental status examination is usually the first assessment completed when people request support or services from a mental health professional. In other areas of clinical practice, a mental status examination is completed when there are reports of alterations in mental well-being. Although this book presents the core components of a psychiatric mental status exam, how the professional gathers this information is an important factor to consider as it affects the validity of the data gathered. For example, when individuals are asked about their experiences they may feel vulnerable, ashamed, or even embarrassed sharing this information. It is the responsibility of the mental health professional to facilitate an engaging relationship with each individual they attempt to assess. The stronger the level of engagement between the professional and the person being assessed, the more likely it is that the assessment information (the content of the psychiatric mental status examination) will accurately reflect current experiences and circumstances. Other factors that affect the outcomes of the assessment are non-verbal and para-verbal cues given by the person being assessed. These cues add another layer of meaning, beyond verbal communication, to the conversation.

The results of a psychiatric mental status examination have three primary purposes: first, to lay the foundation for an effective treatment plan for people experiencing mental health or psychiatric difficulties; second, to capture a person's experience at that moment in time; and third, to be used as a tool to measure change over time. An assessment of a client is the documentation from the mental status examination, which is a method of communicating to other team members.

This book is primarily written with the needs of students, residents, and novice practitioners in mind. The focus is directed toward practical issues related to completing a psychiatric mental status examination. To demonstrate specific teaching points, vignettes and case studies are used to help the reader focus on one aspect of the psychiatric mental status examination at a time. Several chapters conclude with an activity designed to help the reader feel more comfortable with the chapter content. These exercises have been developed to help readers increase their knowledge of each area of the examination. Specific phrases and potential questions that students or novice professionals may use to explore each area of the mental status examination are also provided. An assessment is not complete until it is documented; therefore, ideas on how to effectively document findings within each area of the mental status examination are also shared. The material offered in this book can be used to start thinking about and answering such questions as "How do I get this information?" and "How do I document what I have seen?" The intention is not to present the "right" questions to ask or the "right" way to document responses. The information is presented as an invitation for readers to begin to develop their own interviewing styles and documentation methods. Each professional will develop their own style congruent with their own professional beliefs and practices. Documentation methods will develop based on professional responsibilities and agency policies.

The format of this book provides flexibility; it can be used as a guide for a seminar, in-class activities, or pre- or post-clinical discussions. The book may also be read as a whole or in parts. Each chapter functions as a unit and allows readers to pick and choose relevant material for their particular needs. This book also provides the groundwork to help clinicians develop the skills necessary to effectively assess for potential psychopathology, suicidal or homicidal ideation, and psychosis. This book does not focus on "what" psychopathology, suicidal intent, or psychosis is but instead on how to assess and explore these issues.

Each of the book's 15 chapters focuses on one major content area found in the psychiatric mental status examination and answers a specific question related to completing the examination. For example, the primary purpose of the first chapter is to answer the question, "What is a psychiatric mental status examination?" The second chapter is a starting place for new practitioners, as it helps to clarify the following questions: "What am I looking for?" "When you think about mental health, what image(s) does your mind conjure?" "What would a mental status exam look like if it were completed on a person who was not experiencing symptoms of a mental illness?" In the next 11 chapters, answers are provided to the following questions, as well as many others:

- How is emotional state assessed?
- How is thought content assessed?
- How is speech assessed?
- How are thought process and stream of thought assessed?
- What is a risk assessment?
- How is perception assessed?
- How is a cognitive state or a sensorium assessed?
- How is insight assessed?
- How is volition assessed?
- Why is physical functioning included in a psychiatric mental status exam?

The penultimate chapter explores how to pull all of the information from the preceding chapters together in a meaningful way. The final chapter briefly describes what may happen after the mental status exam is completed.

Each of the chapters from 3 to 13 includes an example of how a specific section of the mental status examination could be documented, special considerations, and lists of terms readers can use as they start to describe the cognitive, affective, and behavioural functioning of their clients. These lists are not comprehensive, but they will give beginning clinicians a place to start as they think about how to document their observations. Many chapters include study questions, a case study with related questions, and an activity to help readers familiarize themselves with the content of each chapter.

The primary purpose of this book is to be a quick and flexible guide that examines the major areas of a comprehensive psychiatric mental status examination. The goal is to stimulate the reader's curiosity about the psychiatric mental status examination. Hopefully, this curiosity will entice readers to continue on a path of discovery and open them to learning about, practising, and completing psychiatric mental status examinations.

# CHAPTER 1

## Psychiatric Mental Status Examination

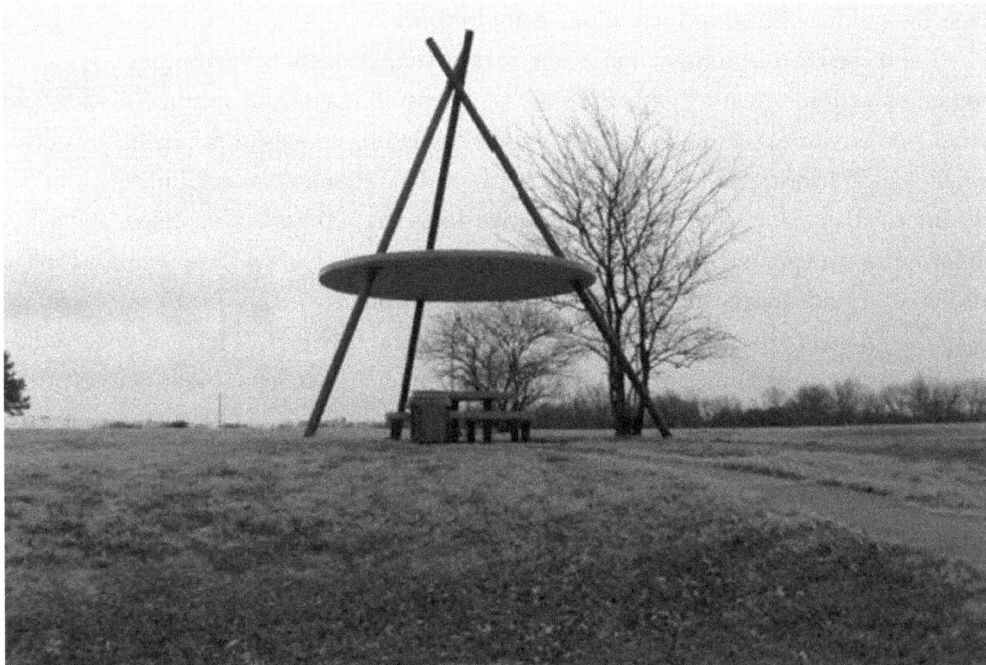

**Photo 1.1:** The Meeting Place

A picture means I know where I was every minute. That's why I take pictures.
It's a visual diary.
   —*Andy Warhol*

## LEARNING OBJECTIVES

**At the completion of this chapter, the reader will be able to:**

- identify the components of a psychiatric mental status examination
- describe who conducts psychiatric mental status examinations
- compare and contrast a relational interview with a non-relational interview
- differentiate key terms used to describe psychiatric mental status examinations

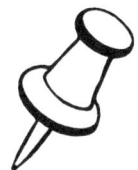

# WHAT IS A PSYCHIATRIC MENTAL STATUS EXAMINATION?

A documented psychiatric mental status examination, sometimes referred to as a mental status exam or simply a mental status, is a means of organizing clinician observations and client experiences about current cognitive, affective, and behavioural functioning. The clinician gathers sufficient data to develop and record a verbal picture of the client: how the person thinks, feels, and acts at one point in time.

The mental status examination is one part of your professional assessment. It can be combined with information gathered from the biopsychosocial and spiritual history, and other auxiliary information from other sources, including friends or family of the client, psychological investigations, and, if indicated, medical examinations. Clinicians can use the information gathered to develop a tentative diagnosis of the client's problem and begin to formulate an appropriate treatment plan. The psychiatric mental status examination is also used to guide diagnostic decisions for clinicians who use the *Diagnostic and Statistical Manual of Mental Disorders* to classify mental disorders. Having this level of understanding also permits the clinician to make a prediction about the most likely course of the person's illness or injury.

Completing a psychiatric mental status exam is much like taking a photograph. Just as a photograph captures people—their expressions, posture, and environment—at a particular point in time, so does a psychiatric mental status exam. We can take another picture or complete another psychiatric mental status exam, but it will never be the same as the first one. Another comparison is an individual's blood pressure reading. The reading reflects their blood pressure only at the time it was measured. The reading does not tell you what their blood pressure was yesterday or what it will be tomorrow.

Additionally, learning about the mental status examination will help clinicians better understand the professional documentation of other health care providers. By becoming familiar with the psychiatric terms used to describe a person's mental state, clinicians will be better able to communicate clearly about client issues and concerns with interdisciplinary team members, which increases team efficiency and improves client safety. Although the mental status examination reports on the presentation of symptoms, rather than etiology, its usefulness is not limited to psychiatry and mental health; it also assists in care planning when symptoms are related to neurological disorders, trauma, metabolic disorders, infectious and parasitic disorders, neoplastic disorders, and so on.

The following pages contain a description of one commonly used format for recording the psychiatric mental status examination. The main sections of a mental status examination typically include the following: general description, emotional state, thought processes, thought content, risk assessment, perception, cognitive state, insight, volition, speech, and physical functioning (see figure 1.1). The chapters that follow describe each

## Components of a Mental Status Exam

| General description | Emotional state | Cognitive state |
| --- | --- | --- |
| Speech | Thought processes | Thought content | Insight |
| Physical functioning | Perception | Risk assessment | Volition |

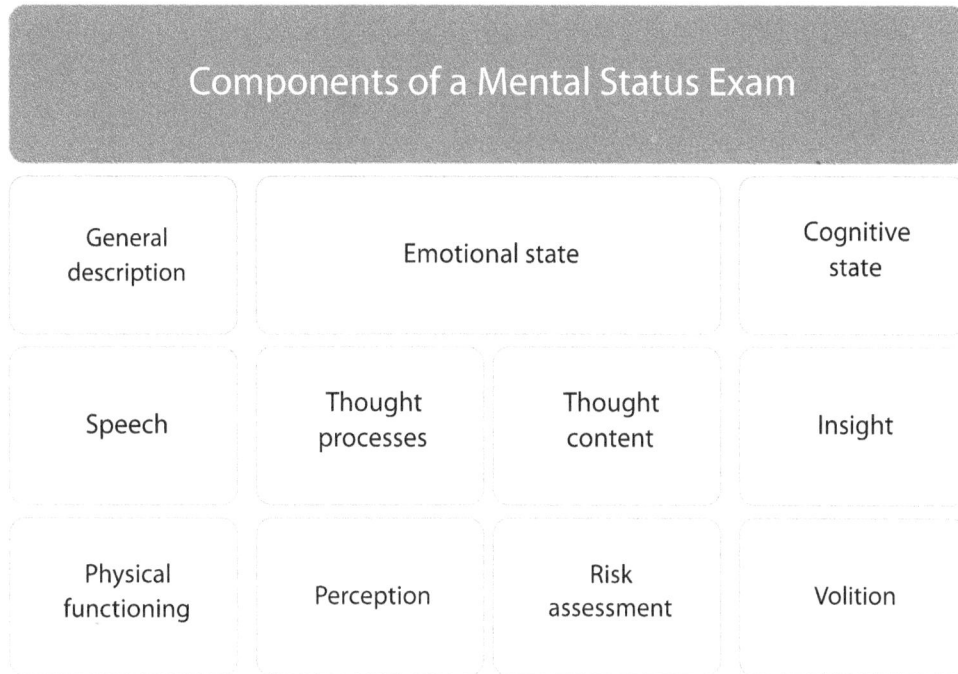

**Figure 1.1:** Main Sections of the Mental Status Examination

of these assessment areas. The categories given here are in no way mutually exclusive, nor does the order in which the various subcomponents listed demand absolute adherence; however, it is easier to start with general description, as this part of the assessment begins as soon as you see the client.

As information is gathered in each of the main areas of the mental status exam, the clinician must be aware that ethnicity, culture, social values, age, personal experiences, and socio-economic factors influence the reliability of the results. Box 1.1 outlines strategies that can be used to reduce clinician biases and prejudices when assessing people from different ethnic, racial, and cultural groups. When determining diagnosis, care plans, or treatment priorities, the results of the mental status exam must be considered along with the individual's personal and family history, and other biological, social, spiritual, and psychological assessments. For example, a person may describe feeling deep and overwhelming sadness. This feeling is consistent with depression, but also with a significant personal loss. The results of the mental status exam alone will not provide the information needed to determine the reason for the sadness. Another example is a person who has performed very poorly on the memory tests within the cognitive state assessment portion of the mental status exam. This poor performance could be related to a number of different issues, including difficulty hearing or understanding the questions, the presence of distractions in the room where the interview is held, language barriers, or a neurocognitive disorder.

## BOX 1.1: REDUCING BIAS AND PREJUDICE

1.  Complete a self-assessment about potential biases and prejudices.

2.  Reflect on the potential effects of acculturation on assessment findings and the development of treatment plans.

3.  Identify and implement strategies that can be used to complete a psychiatric mental status examination in a cultural context.

4.  Identify potential culturally bound mental experiences that are unique to the clinician or person being assessed.

*Source:* Paniagua, F. A. (2010). Assessment and diagnosis in a cultural context. In M. M. Leach & J. D. Aten (Eds.), *Culture and the therapeutic process: A guide for mental health professionals* (pp. 65–98). New York: Routledge.

When completing the mental status examination, the clinician must determine what is a significant finding. When we complete an assessment, what are we expecting? When is something "abnormal"? What are the boundaries between the expected and the unexpected? These questions are the focus of chapter 2. It is important for the clinician to remember that clients who are different (in terms of culture, age, ethnicity, social expectations, or socio-economic status) or who have unexpected findings are not abnormal, deviant, pathological, or problematic—they are simply different than the clinician. When collecting the information needed to complete a mental status examination, the clinician needs to be aware of the biases, potential errors, and other consequences that may arise as a result of these differences (Fontes, 2010). These differences should be documented if they will affect how the care plan is developed and the delivery of treatment.

## WHO CONDUCTS A PSYCHIATRIC MENTAL STATUS EXAMINATION?

Registered nurses, social workers, physicians, psychologists, practical nurses, psychiatric nurses, occupational therapists, physiotherapists, respiratory therapists, recreation therapists, and other health professionals may be required to complete a mental status examination. This examination can occur in many different settings including community health centres, during home care visits, at a health provider's office, in emergency rooms and surgical and medicine units, and in elderly care centres.

Although initially the process of carrying out and recording a psychiatric mental status examination may seem tedious, repetitive, and an inefficient use of time, with practice, the structure that it provides will streamline the recording of clinical data and ensure that important issues are not forgotten, which will result in considerable time savings in the long run.

When using the data gathered from a mental status examination, it is important not to hold the mental status part of the interview in isolation when considering the client's health. When attempting to arrive at a formulation about the individual's current concerns, problems, and difficulties, it is crucial that clinicians synthesize the information derived not only from the mental status exam, but also from the biopsychosocial and spiritual history, information from referrals, and, if indicated, from specialized psychological testing and medical assessments.

It is also important that clinicians guard against interfering with the free flow and spontaneity of an interview by attempting to be too systematic in their observations and questioning the client too much, which may prevent the clinician from interacting with their client in a warm, caring, and genuinely interested way. Too much attention in gathering details for later documentation can make clinicians seem stiff and unresponsive, and can create an air of artificiality in the interview that interferes with the development of the therapeutic relationship. Although several ideas are presented in this book that may help clinicians assess each area of a client's mental status, it is important that clinicians acknowledge each response before moving onto the next section. Box 1.2 provides brief examples of relational and non-relational interviews.

## BOX 1.2: RELATIONAL INTERVIEWING: WHAT IT IS AND IS NOT

Scenario: Jaxxon is brought to the emergency room by his wife. He has been in bed for five days, has stopped eating, and only tells her that he doesn't feel good. Jaxxon has had depression in the past. During the last exacerbation of this depression, his symptoms were treated with a course of electroconvulsive shock treatments. Once these treatments were completed, he began to see a psychiatrist who prescribed antidepressants. He also saw a psychologist for individual psychotherapy.

### What It Is
The following is an excerpt from a conversation Jaxxon had with a clinician in the emergency room who chose to use relational interviewing techniques.

**Clinician:** "What has brought you here today?"
**Jaxxon:** *Sits with his hands folded in his lap, eyes cast downward. He sits silently for one minute and then responds in a low monotone voice.* "My wife says that something is wrong with me."
**Clinician:** "It sounds like she is concerned about you."
**Jaxxon:** "Maybe. I was like this once before."

*continued*

Clinician: "What do you mean?"

Jaxxon: "Feeling numb, and just not having the energy to do anything."

Clinician: "How do you deal with this experience?"

Jaxxon: "I just want to sleep and not wake up."

Clinician: "When you felt like this before, how did you manage these symptoms?"

Jaxxon: "I tried to kill myself. That didn't work out and my wife found me, called the ambulance, and I was taken to the hospital."

Clinician: "Do you have thoughts of harming yourself now?"

Jaxxon: "No. I just want to sleep. My wife says I shouldn't have stopped taking my pills."

### What It Is Not

The following is an excerpt from a conversation Jaxxon had with a clinician in the emergency room who does not use relational interviewing techniques.

Clinician: "What has brought you here today?"

Jaxxon: *Sits with his hands folded in his lap, eyes cast downward. He sits silently for one minute and then responds in a low monotone voice.* "My wife says that something is wrong with me."

Clinician: "Okay, thanks. How would you describe your mood?"

Jaxxon: "I feel nothing."

Clinician: "Do you have thoughts of harming yourself or others?"

Jaxxon: "No—I just want to sleep and not wake up."

Clinician: "So you are not feeling suicidal. Okay."

Jaxxon: "I just feel numb. I have felt numb for the last month."

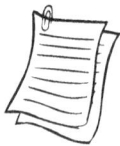

## CHAPTER GLOSSARY TERMS

**affect:** The emotional feeling or tone attached to an object, idea, or thought. This includes inner feelings and their external manifestations.

**anxiety:** An unpleasurable affect consisting of physical changes and a subjective feeling of fear. In contrast to normal fear, the danger or threat in anxiety is unreal. The subjective feeling is an uncomfortable dread of impending danger, accompanied by an overwhelming awareness of being powerless, an inability to perceive the unreality of the threat, a prolonged feeling of tension, and an exhaustive readiness for the expected danger.

**cognition:** The mental process of knowing, thinking, and becoming aware.

**consciousness:** The level of awareness and degree of alertness.

**insight:** Awareness and understanding of one's illness and the symptoms of illness, with or without an awareness of their cause and result.

**mental status:** The organized recording of a psychiatric interview and examination in which the clinician's observations of the client's behaviour and replies to specific questions are carefully documented to give a picture of the client's general health, appearance, speech, form and content of thought, perceptual processes, state of consciousness, cognitive state, insight, and judgment.

**perception:** The reception of many physical stimuli that bombard a person (sights, sounds, feelings, odours, tastes, and so on) and the mental processes where data is organized. Through perception, a person makes sense out of the many stimuli that bombard them.

## ACTIVITY: WHAT DO I SAY NEXT?

This activity provides an opportunity to refresh your communication skills.

Continuing with the conversation between Jaxxon and the emergency room clinician presented in box 1.2, how would you gather information about why Jaxxon stopped taking his pills and if he has experienced any changes in weight, orientation, memory, abstract thinking ability, or judgment? To prioritize your plan of care, you will also need to know what is most important to Jaxxon. How will you find this out?

To complete this activity, you may write out your responses or work with a partner and role play the conversation. If you choose to role play this conversation, one person should take on the role of the clinician while the other takes on the role of Jaxxon.

**Jaxxon:** "No. I just want to sleep. My wife says I shouldn't have stopped taking my pills."

**Clinician:** _____

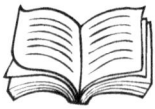

## STUDY QUESTIONS

**1.** What is the primary purpose of conducting a mental status exam?

_____

_____

_____

_____

_____

**2.** Identify two advantages to using psychiatric terminology when documenting a mental status exam.

_____

_____

_____

**3.** What are three important factors that the clinician must consider when they use information gathered during a mental status exam to develop treatment plans?

_____

_____

_____

_____

_____

## REFERENCE

Fontes, L. A. (2010). Considering culture in the clinical intake interview and report. In M. M. Leach & J. D. Aten (Eds.), *Culture and the therapeutic process: A guide for mental health professionals* (pp. 37–64). New York: Routledge.

# CHAPTER 2

## Preparing to Complete a Psychiatric Mental Status Examination

*By Linda Cavanaugh*[1]

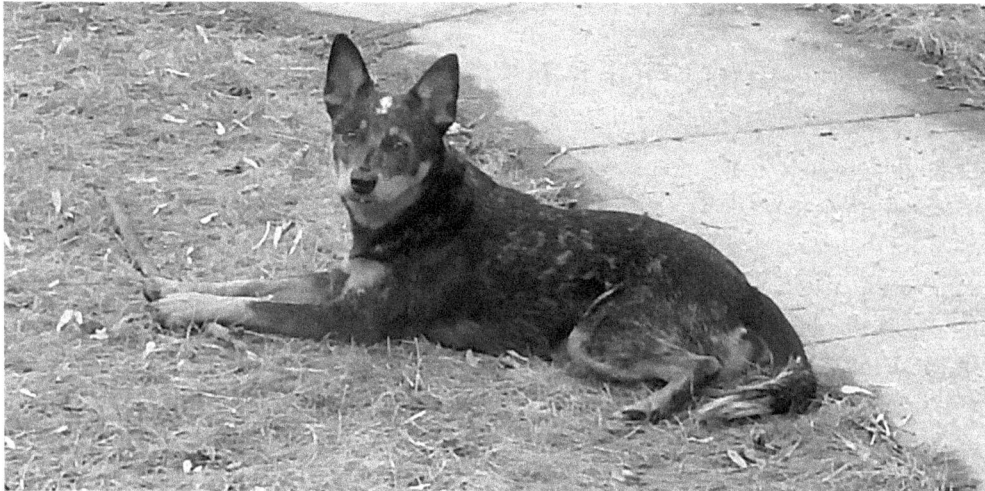

**Photo 2.1:** What Do You See?

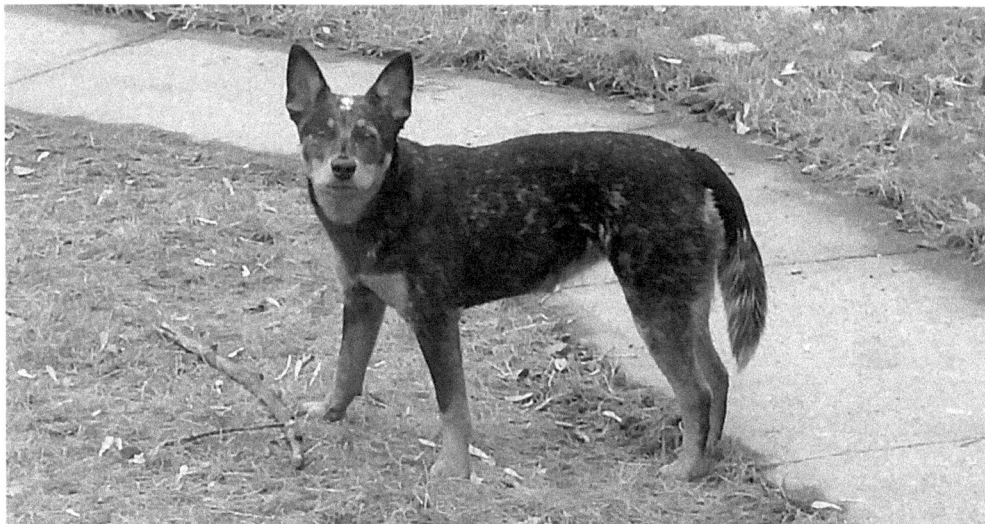

**Photo 2.2:** What Differences Do You See?

> If you don't know what you are looking for, how will you know when you find it?
> —*Anonymous*

# LEARNING OBJECTIVES

**At the completion of this chapter, the reader will be able to:**

- identify personal influences on our beliefs about mental health and mental illness
- describe six categories and indicators of positive mental health
- compare and contrast expected, common variation, and unexpected findings in each of the components of the psychiatric mental status exam

# WHAT ARE YOU LOOKING FOR?

We all have an idea in our minds of what it means and looks like to be mentally "healthy." Before now, you may not have closely examined the image that pops into your mind when you hear the words "mentally healthy." Maybe you have never taken the time to really examine the image in your mind of what mentally "ill" looks like either. Regardless, we all have an image of what it is to be mentally "healthy" or mentally "ill." More often than not those images are influenced by what we see in movies and on social media, what we hear our family and friends say, and our own lived experiences. As a result of these many influences, we have unknowingly compiled an unquestioned image of what it means to be mentally "healthy."

# ACTIVITY: MY IMAGES OF MENTALLY HEALTHY AND MENTALLY ILL

What images of mental health and illness do I have? Take time to ponder and answer the following questions:

- List all of the images and words that come to mind when you think about the idea of "mentally well."

  _____

  _____

  _____

  _____

  _____

- List all of the images and words that come to mind when you think about the idea of "mentally unwell."

  _____

  _____

  _____

  _____

  _____

- List who and what influenced and contributed to your images of mental health.

  _____

  _____

  _____

  _____

  _____

- Are these images accurate?

  _____

  _____

  _____

  _____

  _____

This activity is meant to encourage you to recognize that we are always assessing and comparing the actions, words, and appearances of everyone we meet to some preconceived image we have in our minds of what is "appropriate," "normal," or "ideal." When the person we are assessing does not match our image, we often conclude that something is "wrong," "missing," or "flawed" with that person. Sometimes these conclusions are based on biases and conjecture. As a health professional, these conclusions need to be based on observations and accurate assessments from objective and subjective information.

When assessing the mental health of an individual, it is important to make sure the image we are comparing the person to is accurate, complete, and based in evidence. If we don't, our conclusions are based on nothing more than uninformed opinion.

## WHAT DOES IT MEAN WHEN SOMEONE IS MENTALLY "HEALTHY"?

The World Health Organization (2014) defines mental health as a "state of well-being in which every individual realizes his or her own potential, can cope with the normal stresses of life, can work productively and fruitfully, and is able to make a contribution to her or his community" (p. 1). What is required to achieve this state of well-being and what evidence indicates its presence? It should go without saying, but the first thing necessary for positive mental health is a healthy, physiologically functioning brain. Without the foundation of this healthy organ, the higher functioning skills required for positive mental health will be impacted, in sometimes small and sometimes profound ways. Assuming there is no underlying brain pathology, what do we look for as proof or evidence of positive mental health in an individual?

Marie Jahoda (1958) was the first to classify categories of indicators for positive mental health. She identified attitude toward the self, self-actualization, a unifying outlook on life, autonomy, an accurate perception of reality, and environmental mastery (see box 2.1).

## BOX 2.1: JAHODA'S CATEGORIES AND INDICATORS OF POSITIVE MENTAL HEALTH

1. **Attitudes** of an individual toward his own self (self-acceptance, self-confidence, self-reliance, self-concept, self-esteem)
   a) Ability to display self-acceptance, self-confidence, self-reliance, self-concept, self-esteem

2. **Growth**, development, or self-actualization (motivational processes and the investment in living)
   a) Ability to self-motivate, set and achieve goals
   b) Ability to invest in life such as concern for others, work, ideas, and interests

3. **Integration** (interrelation or balance of psychic forces: ego, superego, id or unconscious, preconscious or conscious) in an individual, a unifying outlook on life (feeling there is a purpose and meaning to life), and resistance to stress (resilience, frustration-tolerance)
   a) Ability to balance conscious, unconscious, and preconscious aspects of the self
   b) Ability to maintain continuity in personality
   c) Ability to display a unifying outlook on life (feeling there is a purpose and meaning to life)
   d) Ability to resist and adapt to stress (resiliency, frustration-tolerance, anxiety tolerance)

4. **Autonomy** (self-control, self-determination, self-respect)
   a) Ability to display self-control
   b) Ability to determine what is best for the self
   c) Ability to make decisions that are best for the self
   d) Ability to respect one's self

5. **Perception** of reality (freedom from the need to distort one's perception of self and environment)
   a) Freedom from the need to distort one's perception of self and environment
   b) Ability to compare reality to wishes and desires—that is, the ability to seek evidence and accept it even if it does not match desires
   c) Ability to empathize with others

6. **Environmental** mastery (ability to love; adequacy in love, work, and play; adequacy in interpersonal relationships; efficiency in meeting situational requirements; capacity for adaption and adjustment; efficiency in problem solving)
   a) Ability to love
   b) Ability to adequately engage in love, work, and play
   c) Ability to adequately engage in interpersonal relationships
   d) Capable of adaptation and adjustment
   e) Capable of efficient problem solving

*Source:* Jahoda, M. (1958). *Current concepts of positive mental health.* New York: Basic Books.

The criteria for mental health have remained relatively consistent for the past 60 years. More recently, Halter and Haase (2014) identified attributes of mental health that included being able to do the following:

- love and experience joy
- deal with conflicting emotions
- live without (undue) fear, guilt, or anxiety
- take responsibility for one's own actions
- control one's own behaviour
- think clearly (problem solve, use good judgment, reason logically, reach insightful conclusions, be creative)
- relate to others (form relationships; have close, loving, adaptive relationships; experience empathy toward others; manage interpersonal conflict constructively)
- attain self-defined spirituality
- negotiate each developmental task
- work and be productive
- maintain a healthy self-concept and self-value
- play and laugh
- accurately appraise reality

Experts in the fields of psychology, social work, nursing, and counselling therapy play an important role in determining the indicators of positive mental health. It is important to note, however, that it is impossible to determine such indicators or qualities of mental health without considering the influence of one's own personal values or beliefs.

# ACTIVITY: TIME TO PONDER

Take time to reflect on and answer the following questions:

- How would you objectively measure the indicators or attributes of mental health listed above? (For example: What constitutes close, loving relationships? How would you measure that? What does being able to work and be productive look like? How would you objectively measure that?)

_____

_____

_____

_____

_____

_____

_____

_____

_____

_____

- How will you be aware of your own personal values when interpreting whether the client displays these indicators or attributes in "positive" or "healthy" ways?

_____

_____

_____

_____

_____

# ASSESSMENT FOR THE "EXPECTED"

Now that you have been able to think about your image of mental health in comparison to expert opinion and evidence, you are ready to begin objectively assessing your client's mental health status. There are several appropriate assessment tools to help you do this. One such fundamental assessment tool is the psychiatric mental status examination, introduced in chapter 1. In psychiatry, this examination is analogous to the physical examination in general medicine. Rather than focusing on biological systems, the mental status examination evaluates an individual's current cognitive, affective (emotional), and behavioural functioning. The mental status examination is a tool that aids in collecting and organizing data about the client's appearance, behaviour, language patterns, mood and affect, thought, perceptions, cognitive ability, and insight and volition.

The following tables will aid in your assessment by showing examples of "expected" findings in mentally healthy clients, as well as common variations or medically related variations, and unexpected findings that may indicate mental health concerns that require further assessment. The information in the tables is not mutually exclusive, as some expected variations may be presented in multiple sections of the mental status examination. Tables 2.1, 2.2, and 2.3 relate to the general description section of the exam. Table 2.4 is specific to the emotional state section. Table 2.5 relates to assessing speech. Table 2.6 focuses on thought processes (also commonly referred to as stream of thought). Table 2.7 pertains to thought content. Table 2.8 is an introductory description of risk assessment comparators. Table 2.9 illustrates aspects of thought perception. Descriptors of cognitive state are provided in table 2.10, while tables 2.11 and 2.12 provide a preliminary introduction to insight and volition. The last table in the chapter, table 2.13, refers to physical functioning. As you begin to learn more about completing the mental status examination, you will be able to add information to each of the tables.

**Table 2.1:** Appearance: Expected Findings, Common Variations, and Findings That Require Further Assessment

| Appearance | Expected findings | Common variations | Further assessment required (unexpected findings) |
|---|---|---|---|
| **Dress/clothing** | Clean, appropriate fit<br><br>Appropriate for age, gender, and situation | Male clothing for female in transition<br><br>Female clothing for male in transition | Dirty, ill-fitting<br><br>Inappropriate for situation |
| **Grooming** | Neat, clean | Teenage trends (e.g., goth, anime)<br><br>Dreadlocks, hair coverings | Dirty, rotten or missing teeth<br><br>Foul body odour |
| **Age** | Physical age matches chronological age | Younger looking due to healthy, active lifestyle | Significantly older looking than chronological age |
| **Height** | Appropriate for age and sex | Genetic predisposition to being unusually tall or short | Significantly shorter than expected in children |
| **Weight** | Appropriate for age and gender | Athletes may weigh less than expected (e.g., marathon runners) or more than expected (e.g., body builders) | Significantly heavier or lighter than expected |
| **Facial expression** | Mirrors expressed thoughts and feelings | Physical impairment may alter facial expression (e.g., stroke, Bell's palsy) | Facial expression is incongruent with expressed thoughts and feelings |

*continued*

| Eye contact | Comfortable eye contact | Cultural variations (e.g., some Indigenous cultures avoid direct eye contact) | Avoids all eye contact

Direct and constant staring |

**Table 2.2:** Behaviour and Motor Activity: Expected Findings, Common Variations, and Findings That Require Further Assessment

| Behaviour and motor activity | Expected findings | Common variations | Further assessment required (unexpected findings) |
|---|---|---|---|
| *Mannerisms* | Habits, gestures, or traits that are minimal and congruent with situation | Nervous laughter | Excessive or inappropriate to situation (e.g., constant finger tapping, rocking back and forth) |
| *Gestures* | Calm, controlled

Matches verbal expression | Cultural variations (e.g., French, talking with hands) | Agitated, erratic, or incongruent with verbal expression |
| *Posture* | Erect and relaxed | Physical limitations (e.g., scoliosis, stroke) | Slumped, hunched, rigid |
| *Position* | Sitting comfortably, arms relaxed at side, head facing speaker | Lying comfortably (e.g., in a hospital bed) | Rigid, fetal position, arms folded over body tightly, head turned away |
| *Gait* | Base width equal to shoulder width; accurate foot placement; smooth, even, and well-balanced walk; presence of associated movements such as symmetrical arm swing | Physical limitations (e.g., stroke, multiple sclerosis, amputation, Parkinson's disease) | Shuffling, stomping, swaying side to side, arms held tight at sides, exaggerated arm swing, staggering |

**Table 2.3:** Attitude: Expected Findings, Common Variations, and Findings That Require Further Assessment

| Attitude during interview | Expected findings | Common variations | Further assessment required (unexpected findings) |
|---|---|---|---|
| *Behaviour based on thoughts or beliefs* | Polite, respectful, calm | Expression of behaviour congruent with thoughts and beliefs | Belligerent, aggressive, terrified, paranoid |

**Table 2.4:** Emotional State: Expected Findings, Common Variations, and Findings That Require Further Assessment

| Emotional state | Expected findings | Common variations | Further assessment required (unexpected findings) |
|---|---|---|---|
| **Mood (a temporary state of mind or feeling)** | Short-lived, appropriate to situation | Grief with loss, anger with injustice, laughter with happiness | Mood incongruent with situation (e.g., happy at a funeral, sad at birth of a baby)<br><br>Sustained mood over a period of time |
| **Affect (observable manifestations of subjectively experienced feelings)** | Smiling, pleasant interaction, comfortable, co-operative | Manifestations appropriate to mood (e.g., crying when sad) | Manifestations inappropriate to stated mood (flat, slumped body position, distrustful, suspicious) |
| **Anxiety** | None | Slightly anxious in unfamiliar surroundings or situations | Uncontrolled panic, excessive fear for situation |

**Table 2.5:** Speech: Expected Findings, Common Variations, and Findings That Require Further Assessment

| Speech | Expected findings | Common variations | Further assessment required (unexpected findings) |
|---|---|---|---|
| **Volume** | Moderate | Dysarthria related to medical diagnosis<br><br>Dysphonia related to medical diagnosis | Loud, yelling, whisper, mute |
| **Rate** | Unhurried, fluent stream, even pace | Rate matches heightened emotion (e.g., fast when anxious, slow when confused)<br><br>Dysarthria<br><br>Dysphonia | Stutter, rapid, continuous stream without pause or breath |
| **Quality** | Word choice appropriate to culture and education | Word choice and sentence structure are awkward (English is a second language) | Word choice inappropriate to culture and education |
| **Comprehension** | Understands speech, able to identify when unable to understand words | Aphasia with stroke | Does not understand simple speech<br><br>Gives inappropriate meaning to words |
| **Clarity** | Clear articulation | Dysarthria<br><br>Dysphonia | Garbled, monotone |

**Table 2.6:** Thought Processes (Stream of Thought): Expected Findings, Common Variations, and Findings That Require Further Assessment

| Thought process (also known as stream of thought) | Expected findings | Common variations | Further assessment required (unexpected findings) |
|---|---|---|---|
| *Rate of thought (the speed of thinking)* | Timely response to conversation flow | Slowed thinking due to extreme fatigue<br><br>Processing speed slows with the onset of neurocognitive diseases | Delayed response, rushed response<br><br>Does not wait for others to finish their thoughts or sentences |
| *Flow of ideas (the amount of thoughts)* | Completes one idea before moving on to another idea | Drug side effects | Moves quickly from one topic to another before completing the first train of thought<br><br>Persistent and inappropriate repetition of the same thoughts |
| *Form of thought (the way we link ideas together)* | Logical, goal directed, coherent, relevant | Drug interactions | Concepts and things are grouped together that are not closely connected<br><br>Illogical, general lack of clarity, tangential |

**Table 2.7:** Thought Content: Expected Findings, Common Variations, and Findings That Require Further Assessment

| Thought content | Expected findings | Common variations | Further assessment required (unexpected findings) |
|---|---|---|---|
| *Thought content* | Consistent and logical | The parents of a child who is immuno-compromised may worry about germs or contamination | Belief that people are out to get them<br><br>Sense of over importance about themselves<br><br>Belief that others can hear their thoughts<br><br>Worries about germs or contamination |

**Table 2.8:** Risk Assessment: Expected Findings, Common Variations, and Findings That Require Further Assessment

| Risk assessment | Expected findings | Common variations | Further assessment required (unexpected findings) |
|---|---|---|---|
| *Suicidal/homicidal thoughts* | None | A person with uncontrollable pain or an incurable illness may wonder if death is a better option than living in their current state | Thoughts of self-harm; thoughts of harming others; plan for either suicide or homicide |

**Table 2.9:** Perception: Expected Findings, Common Variations, and Findings That Require Further Assessment

| Perception | Expected findings | Common variations | Further assessment required (unexpected findings) |
|---|---|---|---|
| *Hallucination* | None | Drug interactions/delirium | Auditory/visual hallucinations |
| *Misidentification* | None | Later stages of neurocognitive diseases | People known as familiar are seen as unfamiliar |
| | | | People known as unfamiliar are seen as familiar |
| *Depersonalization* | None | Extreme fatigue | Feeling detached from oneself; feeling "mechanical" |

**Table 2.10:** Cognitive State: Expected Findings, Common Variations, and Findings That Require Further Assessment

| Cognitive state | Expected findings | Common variations | Further assessment required (unexpected findings) |
|---|---|---|---|
| *Consciousness* | Awake and alert, aware of stimuli from environment and within the self and responds appropriately to stimuli | There may be several underlying medical causes | Confused, unresponsive, stupor, lethargy |
| *Orientation* | Oriented to person, place, and time | Brain injury, neurocognitive diseases, drug side effects | Disorientation |

*continued*

| | | | |
|---|---|---|---|
| ***Concentration and attention*** | Completes thoughts without wandering<br><br>Pays attention to people and sur-roundings without distraction | Drug interactions | Difficulty staying with conversation<br><br>Easily distracted<br><br>Irrelevant replies or comments to conversation |
| ***General information*** | Aware of common cur-rent events, aware of well-known facts (e.g., names of provinces, prime minister) | New to country, city, or province | Unable to identify or discuss well-known events or facts |
| ***Intellectual ability/ intelligence*** | Problem-solving and reasoning abilities match general intelli-gence level | Unfamiliarity with language, unable to hear all components of questions | Unable to problem solve or reason at a level expected for age, education, and life experience |
| ***Memory*** | Appropriate short- and long-term memory recall | Fatigue<br><br>Pain<br><br>Drugs<br><br>Underlying medical conditions | Unable to recall recent events<br><br>Unable to remember significant past events |
| ***Judgment*** | Able to explain deci-sions with appropriate rationale | Drugs, lack of understanding | Impulsive or inappropriate decision making |
| ***Abstract thinking*** | Able to discuss common concepts | Consider growth and development stages (e.g., Piaget) | Unable to distinguish between con-nected concepts (lazy versus idle) |

**Table 2.11:** Insight: Expected Findings, Common Variations, and Findings That Require Further Assessment

| Insight | Expected findings | Common variations | Further assessment required (unexpected findings) |
|---|---|---|---|
| ***Insight*** | Provides clear ration-ale for choices and decisions | Strong beliefs (e.g., religious) form the basis of all deci-sions regardless of consequences | Unable to provide clear explanations for choices and decisions |

**Table 2.12:** Volition: Expected Findings, Common Variations, and Findings That Require Further Assessment

| Volition | Expected findings | Common variations | Further assessment required (unexpected findings) |
|---|---|---|---|
| *Volition (will)* | Ability to make a conscious choice or decision | Drug side effects or interactions | Excessively indecisive<br><br>Unable to choose<br><br>Unable to identify options in decision making |

**Table 2.13:** Physical Functioning: Expected Findings, Common Variations, and Findings That Require Further Assessment

| Physical functioning | Expected findings | Common variations | Further assessment required (unexpected findings) |
|---|---|---|---|
| *Physical functioning* | Intact physical structure and function | Rule out physiological/biological causes of mental health symptoms (e.g., brain tumours, drug interactions) | Impaired physical structure or function resulting in mental health symptoms |

# CHAPTER GLOSSARY TERMS

**facial expression:** The positioning of one's facial muscles that is often used to convey a feeling.

**gait:** The manner in which a person walks.

**gesture:** The movement of a body part to convey an idea or a feeling.

**grooming:** The activity of tending to one's appearance and hygiene.

**mannerisms:** Are seen in most people, are not as persistent as stereotypes, and are more in keeping with the individual's personality. They are more frequently in evidence in people under some stress. Examples include shoulder shrugging, repeatedly clearing the throat, and blinking.

**position:** The particular way a person places or arranges their body.

**posture:** The position in which someone holds their body.

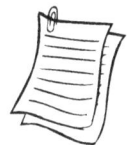

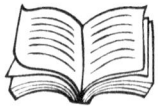

# STUDY QUESTIONS

**1.** How do we form our own images of mental health and mental illness?

_____

_____

_____

_____

_____

**2.** Based on the World Health Organization's definition of mental health, what four essential abilities must a person have in order to be considered mentally healthy?

_____

_____

_____

_____

_____

**3.** What are Jahoda's six categories of positive mental health?

_____

_____

_____

_____

_____

_____

_____

_____

_____

_____

_____

# NOTE

1.  Linda Cavanaugh, RN, BScN, MAd, ED, is an assistant professor at MacEwan University who has many years of experience teaching novice health care students. When I started writing this book it was intended to be a resource for beginning practitioners. Linda insightfully asked me, "How are people supposed to recognize different than expected, if they don't know what is expected?" Recognizing that this was an essential feature that was missed in many resources in this area, Linda generously gave her time and energy to develop this chapter, which helps to contextualize the other chapters in this workbook.

# REFERENCES

Halter, M. J., & Haase, M. (2014). Mental health and mental illness. In C. Pollard, S. Ray, & M. Haase (Eds.), *Varcarolis's Canadian Psychiatric Mental Health Nursing: A Clinical Approach* (1st Canadian ed.) (pp. 2–16). Toronto: Elsevier Canada.

Jahoda, M. (1958). *Current concepts of positive mental health*. New York: Basic Books.

World Health Organization. (2014). *Mental health: A state of wellbeing*. Retrieved from http://www. who.int/features/factfiles/mental_health/en/

# CHAPTER 3

## General Description

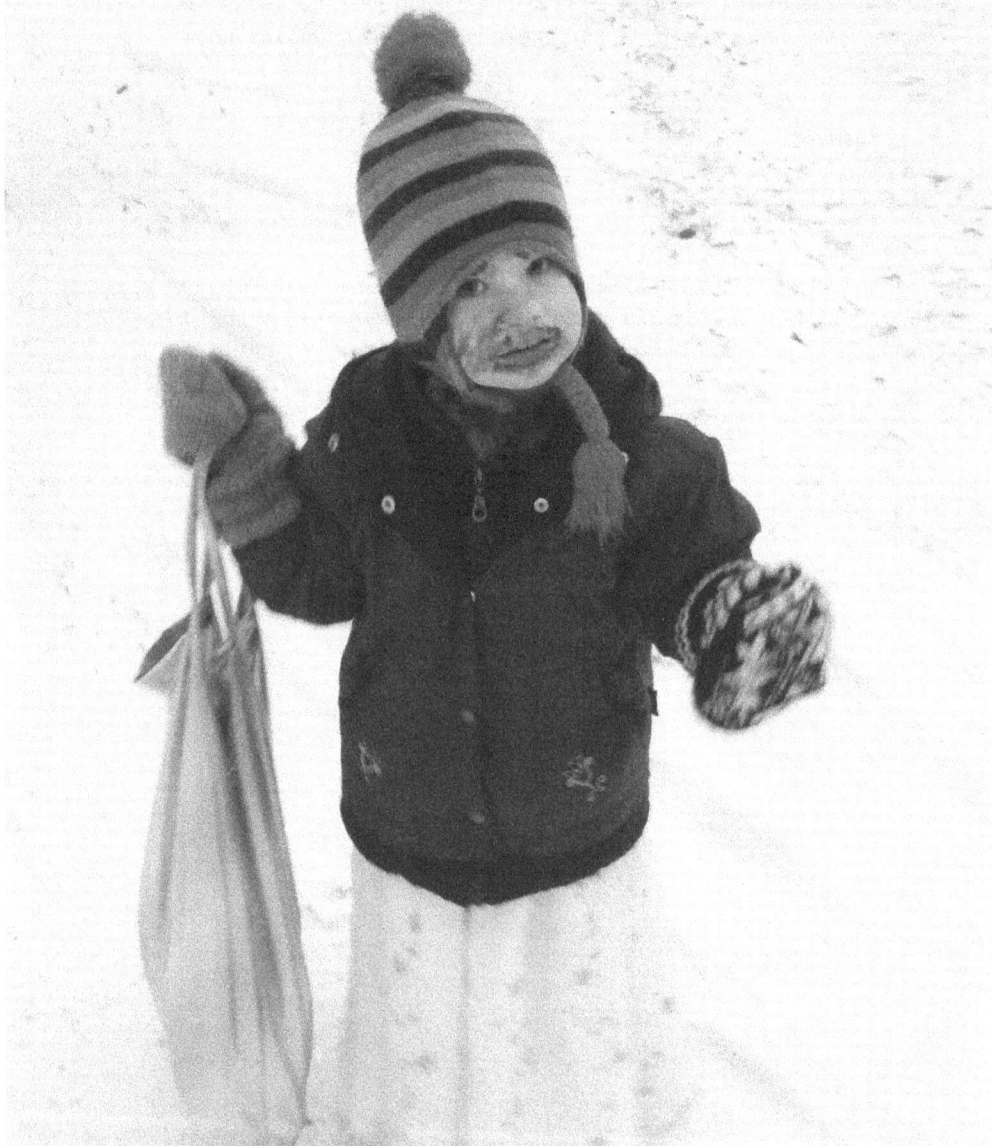

**Photo 3.1:** Winter Princess

Everyone sees what you appear to be, few experience what you really are.
—*Niccolò Machiavelli,* The Prince

# LEARNING OBJECTIVES

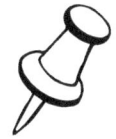

**At the completion of this chapter, the reader will be able to:**

- identify the major categories within the general description component of the psychiatric mental status exam
- describe assessment indicators for appearance, behaviour and motor activity, and attitude
- document assessment findings using objective observations
- define key terms that may be used in this section of the psychiatric mental status examination
- discuss the importance of objectivity when completing this section of the psychiatric mental status examination

# GENERAL DESCRIPTION: HOW IS THIS ASSESSED?

As completely and accurately as possible, the clinician must summarize observations about the person being assessed. It is imperative that the clinician documents this information in an objective and non-judgmental manner. The appearance of the person being assessed may give clues to his or her underlying illness(es); however, this is only one piece of the assessment. When appearance is taken alone it can be easily misinterpreted and can be prone to bias. Figure 3.1 presents the major headings that can be used to organize the clinician's observations.

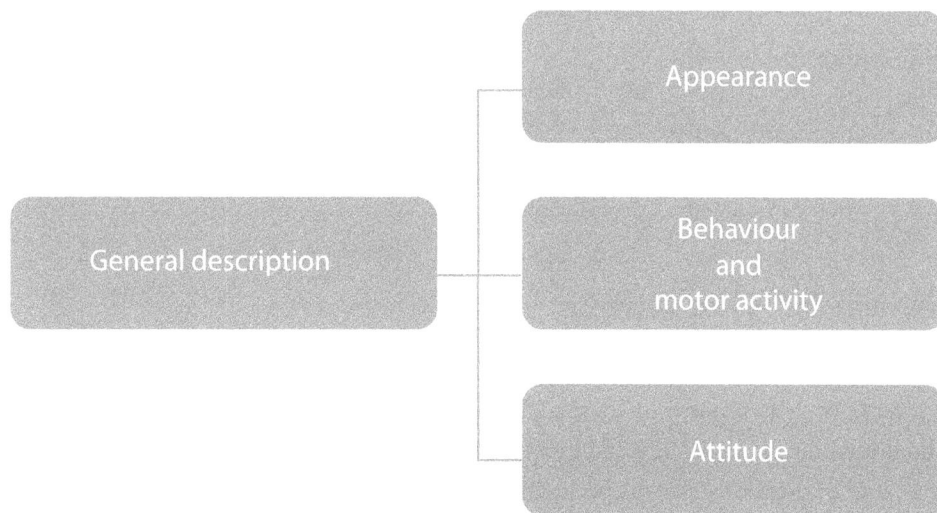

**Figure 3.1:** General Description—Major Categories

## Appearance

As soon as the clinician sees the client the assessment begins. The clinician's observations of the client should include a description of their dress and grooming, physical appearance, facial expression, and eye contact. Box 3.1 provides more information on the indicators within each of these categories.

## BOX 3.1: INDICATORS OF APPEARANCE

Client's dress and grooming:

- inconsistent with season or time of day
- meticulous
- level of hygiene
- unique application of clothing or makeup

Features of physical appearance:

- apparent age in relation to chronological age
- approximate weight and height
- body modifications
- emaciation

Facial expression:

- relationship to expressed mood or thought content

Eye contact:

- avoids eye contact
- stares directly into examiner's eyes

## Behaviour and Motor Activity

Under this heading, the clinician describes the non-verbal behaviour that occurs during the interview. It is important to specifically describe the behaviour or motor activity without attributing it to a specific cause. Details of a person's posture, mobility, movements, and expressions should be identified. Box 3.2 provides a more detailed list of types of behaviours and motor activity a clinician should look for in this part of the mental status exam.

## BOX 3.2: EXAMPLES OF BEHAVIOURS AND MOTOR ACTIVITIES

- mannerisms
- tics
- gestures
- tremors
- restlessness
- slowed responses
- automatic behaviour
- doubled over to relieve pain
- fully ambulatory
- echopraxia (client's body movements copy the interviewer's)
- abnormal breathing patterns (e.g., panting or frog breathing)
- unsteady gait
- walks with assistance
- in a wheelchair
- bedridden

## Attitude During the Interview

Under this heading, the clinician should describe the person's prevailing attitude toward the clinician and toward the experience of being interviewed. The use of adjectives is helpful when documenting information in this section. For example, a person may not have strong feelings about the interview, which may be described as being neutral. The person may display little or no feeling when relating their story or replying to questions, or they may be irritated about the interview. Perhaps this person agreed to come to the interview only at the insistence of a family member. Table 3.1 identifies several examples of positive and negative attitudes that could be displayed during an interview.

**Table 3.1:** Examples of Attitudes That May Be Displayed During an Interview

| Positive attitudes | Negative attitudes |
| --- | --- |
| Determined | Completely unresponsive |
| Motivated | Evasive |
| Interested | Fearful |
| Self-confident | Hostile |
| Self-disciplined | Indecisive |
| Candid | Guarded |
| Humble | Controlling |

People can also demonstrate a different attitude toward the examiner than toward the interview itself. An individual may behave toward the examiner in the following ways:

- friendly
- belligerent
- ingratiating
- sarcastic
- demanding
- pleasant
- flirtatious

Any change in attitude during the course of the interview should be documented. It should be noted whether these changes are gradual or occur in response to specific questions, topics, or circumstances. Additionally, the level of rapport between the client and examiner should also be documented. Box 3.3 explains the types of rapport the examiner may document.

## BOX 3.3: DOCUMENTING GENERAL DESCRIPTION FINDINGS

When documenting what you see, it is important that you describe what you observe in the client. Do not interpret what you are seeing. For example, you may see a number of facial tics during the interview. Write that several facial tics were observed. Do not write that the person has Tourette's, as this would be an interpretation of the cause of the tics. The mental status exam is a "snapshot"— it simply describes, nothing more. Following are two examples of documented general descriptions.

### Georgi
Georgi was a neatly dressed male who was friendly and co-operative during the interview. When invited into the interview room, he independently positioned himself comfortably in the chair and maintained eye contact when responding to questions.

### Alex
Alex is a 17-year-old male, who appears to be older than his stated age. Although it was 24 degrees Celsius on the day of the interview, he wore a heavy winter jacket and ski pants. He frequently scanned the room. He seemed restless, as he frequently repositioned himself in the chair. When he responded to questions, he rarely provided a direct response and at times seemed irritated.

# SPECIAL CONSIDERATIONS

When completing a general description, it is important that the clinician remain objective. Assessments related to appearance and mannerisms must be made within the cultural context of the person being interviewed. When describing the general appearance and attitude of children or adolescents, the clinician must take into account their age.

# CHAPTER GLOSSARY TERMS

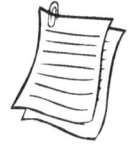

**general description:** The overall appearance of the client, including posture, dress, personal care, hygiene, weight, bearing, movement, and facial expression.

## Appearance

**appropriate:** Clothing worn is suitable for the ensuing activity or environment.
**bizarre:** Unconventional, characterized by strange or eccentric mannerisms, dress, ideas, behaviours, or acts.
**neglected:** Dress and personal hygiene that indicate that the client is either incapable of or has disregarded their self-care.
**unkempt:** Dishevelled, inattentive to personal appearance or hygiene.

## Behaviour and Psychomotor Activity

**affective interaction:** Behaviour during an interview that is emotionally charged.
**aggressive:** Forceful behaviour, whether verbal or physical. It is the motor counterpart to the affect of anger or hostility.
**agitation:** Restless, volatile, or erratic emotional behaviour accompanied by a great deal of motor restlessness and often anxiety.
**akinesia:** A lack of physical movement.
**appropriate:** Behaviour is suited to the requirements of the prevailing situation.
**assaultive:** Physically aggressive and threatening, striking out at others.
**automatic obedience:** A pathological degree of compliance with the instructions of the examiner.
**bizarre:** Unconventional, characterized by strange or eccentric mannerisms, dress, ideas, behaviours, or acts.
**cataleptic:** Condition in which the person maintains the body position into which they are placed.

**compulsive movements:** The result of an irresistible urge to perform a certain act. For example, an uncontrollable need to continually wash one's hands.

**coordinated:** Movements exhibit a normal degree of flexibility and harmony with no sign of impaired motor control.

**decreased interest:** Intellectual behaviour that shows signs of diminishing awareness of, response to, or concern about others, employment, activities, and surroundings; this is indicative of varying degrees of recession into a state of mental and emotional detachment.

**dystonic:** A motor disturbance usually observed as a side effect of phenothiazine drugs and major tranquilizers that consists of uncoordinated and spasmodic movements of the body and limbs, such as arching of the back and twisting of the body and neck.

**echopraxia:** Imitation of another person's movements.

**hysterical:** Behaviour that is marked by excitable, emotional outbursts.

**mannerisms:** Are seen in most people, are not as persistent as stereotypes, and are more in keeping with the person's personality. They are more frequently in evidence in people under some stress. Examples include shoulder shrugging, repeatedly clearing the throat, and blinking.

**negativism:** Opposition to the suggestions of the interviewer to behave in a certain fashion.

**overactive:** Excessive motor activity.

**pacing:** Restlessness characterized by continual walking.

**regressive:** Going back to a more infantile or immature level.

**restless:** Unsettled, fidgety, wandering, agitated.

**retarded:** Movements are slow, laboured, and limited.

**rigid:** Gait and other movements appear stiff and puppet-like, which is indicative of a severe lack of flexibility.

**self-abusive:** Self-inflicted punishment and injury and acts of violence against one's self.

**startle reaction:** Reflex motor response to a sudden, intense stimulus associated with a sudden increase in the level of consciousness. This can occur in anyone in an acute anxiety state.

**stereotypy:** A repetition of the motor action as is seen in chronic schizophrenic states. At times, it is highly organized and appears to be a ritualistic act.

**stuperose:** Lethargy in which the client is immobile, out of touch with their surroundings, and exhibits little or no response to stimuli.

**tantrums:** Uncontrolled, angry outbursts of bad temper.

**tic:** Involuntary, spasmodic, repetitive motor movements of a small segment of the body.

**tremulous:** Movements that indicate impaired motor coordination, ranging from fine muscular tremors to spontaneous, spasmodic jerking.

**withdrawing:** Moving away from or retreating.

## Attitude Toward the Examiner

**aloof:** Distant; emotionally uninvolved.

**belligerent:** Combative, quarrelsome, argumentative, hostile, defiant.

**bored:** Mild degree of emotional detachment indicated by little interest being shown in the conversation or activity, and by signs of weariness and indifference to the activity.

**complaintive:** Given to complaining, blaming, or being overly critical.

**defensive:** Tendency to rationalize or make excuses.

**demanding:** Persistently requiring attention.

**dependent:** Tendency to look to others for emotional support, to require constant reassurance and direction, and to cling.

**evasive:** Rationalizes behaviour, evades or disowns responsibility, and covers up.

**flirtatious:** Seductive and sexually playful.

**inattentive:** Indifferent and lacks interest.

**indifference:** Lacks interest in and concern about the conversation.

**initiates:** Spontaneously begins a conversation in response.

**irritable:** Short-tempered, easily angered or upset, and impatient, with a low frustration tolerance.

**jocular:** Playful, joking interaction.

**overbearing:** Evincing a superior attitude, domineering, arrogant, proud, regarding others with disdain and as inferior, monopolizing.

**pleasant:** Agreeable or harmonious.

**responsive:** Does not initiate conversation but will respond on approach.

**self-centred:** Primarily concerned with one's own desires and needs, and indifferent to those of others.

**suspicious:** Distrustful and accusatory.

**uncommunicative:** Unwilling or unable to verbalize.

# ACTIVITY: GENERAL DESCRIPTION WORD SEARCH

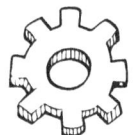

The word search on the following page will help you to familiarize yourself with some of the terms that are often used when documenting assessment findings.

```
V X U H U S S E N S U O I C S N O C O M O T O S E P H J P A R I
Y E N O I T A T N E I R O F J T Q A E S F O K G E Y L M F F Y Z
A I B P C P G X U R W Y Q F A I I R Q R A B E L I T S O H E J H
S U O I T A T R I L F I M Z I D X H S L Y R R X O W Z Q D I I P
B L M I S I D E N T I F I C A T I O N C E Z C N P G Q W T F N R
W X E E I G C B P F C N W D F I T F E C N A R A E P P A G I G O
Z S C E V B G S A H H Y P E R P H A G I A G S D S I F L N D R N
C B H Y P E R M N E S I A S Y T I R A L C D R D E T A T I G A F
P E R S P I R I N G A X M P S T U P O R O S E A E P I L N E N V
E W N E J E N E N C J M P O T T L W D B K F C F N L M C S T D O
R I P K F J R G S S B U I N U J I A I U S K G M E D I N Z I I F
S L F P D E V P K T I J E D T B S A J N S E T N D N E R C N O F
O D Q Q M Q R C L S L G O E T J S B T S D R S E I T S U I G S X
N E G L E C T E D E F E H N E U V U P Z S I L S I L R I R U E I
T R A Z W R Y V N W X M S T R X C H J H X U F O I E B I V S M H
R E I N E O L H F C W E P S I X E W Y W S N M F D O F M A E A O
O D T P I L G A T L E O D C N P X Q Z I O C E Z E Y N P U A A K
T C Y P L M M E P A S S Z K G Y I H O I H O L G P R B C T M W Z
B H C L S L A O T T P M U M I R L N T V Q N A A R X E I X B E O
Z E E O D P L T U D I A M S W N S A N Q G F N O E O C N Y I F X
S Q H S L H N R E C A L L E P H Z L P M G A C H S T H C T V J R
P B Q A J A E V E D R X B Z M I A T J J H B H J S R O O A A R N
L F C B V X I N Y P B X H E L I C Y O A V U O J E K P N O L W Q
I E A P V I O N T I G I G A T S R I O P L L L D Y R G Q E X J
E L A F V I O B M E M R N N L M X V O E U A I G L I A R N N P U
F L R T T K D U S O L O A U Y L E R G U X T C E G C X U Y T E D
T O I I I W L T R R S T R K L R U W O B S I N G L M I E S V R G
H D L O L N U U A R S R I D A V E C P O S O U U L L A N W P S E
R O A E J R G I E M I S E B O R E D I V L N F H N Y K T K U E M
V I B M E N R P U N E R U P W H K O P N N R D T E P T C Y C V E
O N I S U O E C G X D N R L Y S J B D O A E E Z L Q A S Q I E N
L F L B H D R X X E D E J I N H H J I E T T J G E Y W Q S N R T
U I E P F I I A M A B O S O T F Z S F E T B I Z H O P U T O A Y
M D U H C Q C E N E P S I P X A L P L V I A V O R D O U B T T S
E E N O Y U N C G J M S B C A U B B A I T Q M D N L Q H I S I U
V L K B Q T E C T N U O M L P I L L T S U V G I U S A L P Y O R
E I E I I W T R E L A N R M D T R X E A D Z L M N G K J Z D N Z
O T P A Z Y B I L B J X O Y L F M E I V E Q E Z D A K P N X L Y
T Y T I M E X I R O E C O N T R O L W E D R A M A T I C X Q S B
Q A C U N Q N A T W F X W C N J S V M O T O R A C T I V I T Y C
```

**Figure 3.2:** Mental Status Word Search—Recalling Words Related to Assessing General Description

Find the words listed below.

- appearance
- attitude
- behaviour
- despondent
- dramatic
- drowsy

- evasive
- fearful
- fidgeting
- flirtatious
- gestures
- hostile

- neglected
- restless
- sarcastic
- tense
- tics

## STUDY QUESTIONS

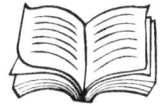

**1.** What are the three major assessment areas within the general description segment of the mental status exam?

_____

_____

_____

**2.** When does the clinician begin to complete the general description?

_____

_____

**3.** How do clinicians ensure that they are documenting their findings in an objective manner?

_____

_____

_____

_____

_____

## CASE STUDY

Misty has just started her mental health clinical rotation. She has been assigned to work with Alex and begins the day by completing the general description portion of the psychiatric mental status examination. She has documented the following:

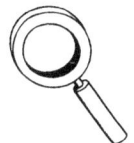

Alex is a teenager who has a real baby face. He states that people often think that he is 13 or 14. His manner of dress is inappropriate and he seems paranoid. He is experiencing psychomotor side effects of his medication. There is a foul odour coming from his body.

## Case Study Questions

What feedback would you give Misty about her documentation?

**1.** What did she do well?

_____
_____
_____
_____

**2.** What could be improved?

_____
_____
_____
_____

**3.** Why should she improve her documentation?

_____
_____
_____
_____

**4.** How could she improve her documentation?

_____
_____
_____
_____

# CHAPTER 4

## Emotional State

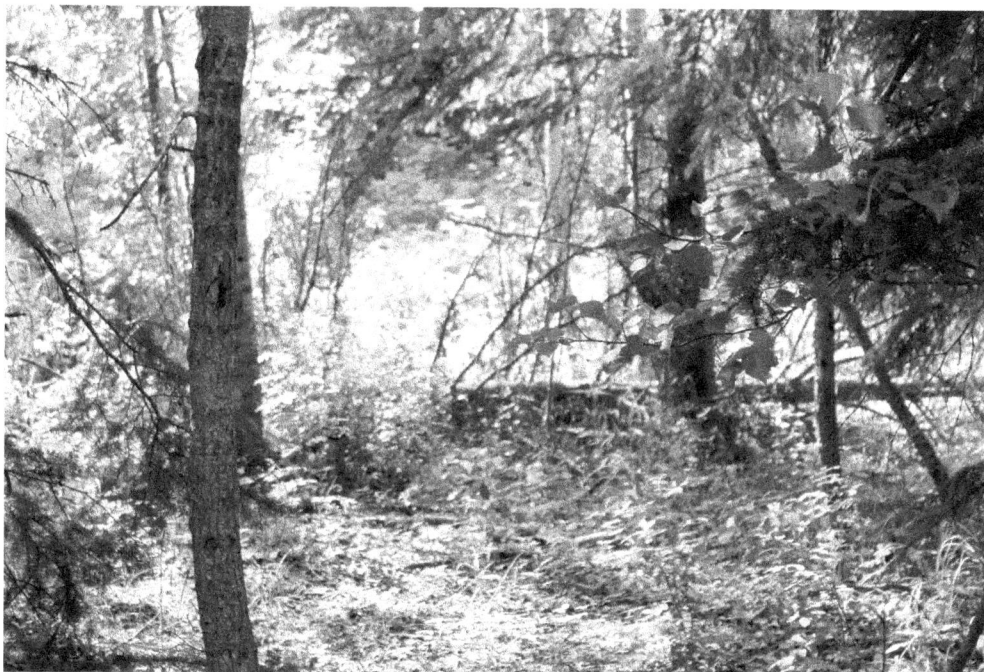

**Photo 4.1:** Deep in the Woods

> When dealing with people, remember you are not dealing with creatures of
> logic, but creatures of emotion.
> —*Dale Carnegie*

## LEARNING OBJECTIVES

**At the completion of this chapter, the reader will be able to:**

- identify the major categories within the emotional state component of the psychiatric mental status examination
- describe assessment indicators for mood and affect
- document objective and subjective assessment findings

- define key terms that may be used in this section of the psychiatric mental status examination
- identify how culture and age may affect the assessment of mood and affect

# HOW IS EMOTIONAL STATE ASSESSED?

The emotional responses of the client are the most difficult part of the mental status to gauge. The technical term for the emotional tone of the client is *affect*. Affects are related to temperamental and developmental factors, and unconscious mental processes. There are two main categories in this section of the mental status: mood and affect.

## Mood

In this section, how the client feels is recorded. It is the person's subjective account of their mood in terms of depth, intensity, duration, reactivity, and stability. The client may use rather non-specific terms to describe their mood. The following are examples of non-specific terms: depressed, hyper, irritable, panicky, terrified, angry, enraged, elated, euphoric, empty, guilty, hopeless, helpless, futile, self-contemptuous, and tense. If any of these descriptors is used by the client, the clinician should attempt to elicit what that word means to the individual. The clinician could ask, "How long have you felt like this?" or "On a scale of one to ten, with one being the worst you could ever imagine feeling, how would you rate the intensity of your mood?"

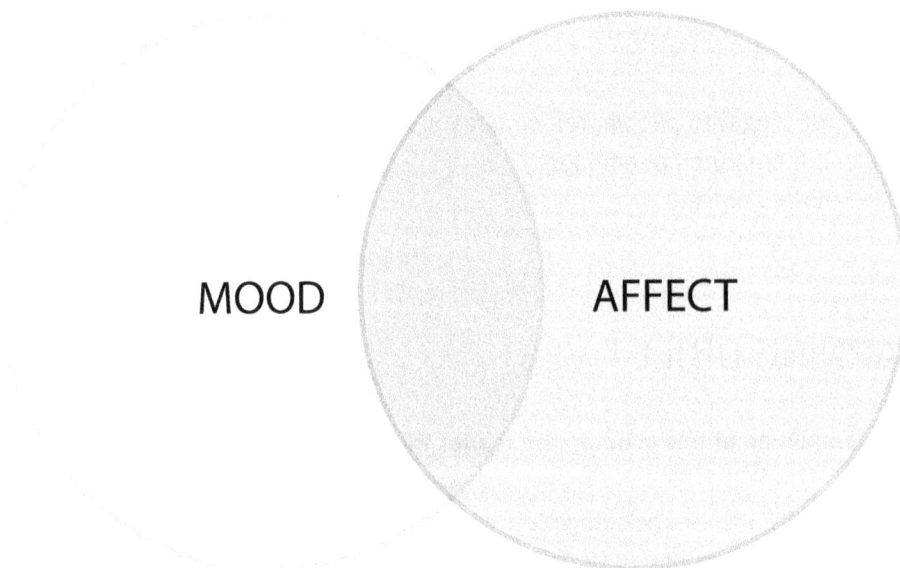

MOOD                    AFFECT

**Figure 4.1:** Emotional State Assessment Areas

## Affect

Under this heading, clinicians record their observations and assessment of the client's prevailing mood or moods. This combines observations of the client's facial expressions, gestures, speed of psychomotor response, and a subjective evaluation of the content of the client's description of themself. It is the clinician who determines a client's affect. Box 4.1 provides examples of terms used to describe affect.

### BOX 4.1: EXAMPLES OF TERMS USED TO DESCRIBE AFFECT

- agitated
- bewildered
- blunted
- constricted
- despondent
- dramatic
- exaggerated
- fixed
- flat
- grandiose
- heightened
- incongruent
- irritable
- labile
- lonely
- non-reactive
- non-responsive
- reactive
- restricted range
- suspicious

Documentation of affect includes range, change in pattern, intensity, and appropriateness. Appropriateness of affect is determined by comparing emotional expression to the content of what the client is thinking or speaking. Clinicians determine affect to be appropriate if the emotional expression and what the client is describing are congruent. For example, a young person with schizophrenia recounts the death of her father, laughing and giggling during her account, which indicates inappropriateness or incongruous affect. The constancy of the affect during the interview should be attended to, and the influences that change the affect during the interview should be noted. Box 4.2 provides examples of documentation of affect.

## BOX 4.2: DOCUMENTING EMOTIONAL STATE

### Congruence

She describes her mood as sad and feels like everyone is against her. If she could, she would like to crawl into a hole and not move. She gets angry at times—however, not at her children. There are no experiences of anxiety reported. Her affect is congruent with her mood.

### Non-congruence

Outwardly he appeared calm and relaxed; however, he described experiencing significant amounts of tension and worry in his life.

# SPECIAL CONSIDERATIONS

When assessing a person's emotional state, it is important to consider both recent and past events when determining if there is congruent affect. For example, determining how long a person can be expected to grieve or isolate themselves after a death of a loved one will affect how the results of an emotional assessment need to be interpreted. These results must be communicated to other team members with supporting information related to the cultural context of the assessment. Additionally, experiences of loss and grief can vary significantly among individuals. Beginning clinicians will want to seek support from an experienced mentor as they make a determination of whether the assessment findings are expected, unexpected, or represent a common variation.

A clinician must also demonstrate a great deal of thoughtfulness when assessing the emotional state of children. Children may not have the words to accurately describe their mood. They may not understand what is meant by mood. Box 4.3 provides additional statements and questions that can be used during an emotional assessment of a child. A faces chart (see photo 4.2) can also be used to help younger children communicate how they feel.

## BOX 4.3: ASSESSING THE EMOTIONAL STATE OF CHILDREN

The following statements and questions can be used to help assess the emotional state of children:

- Tell me about the last time you felt happy.
- How often do you cry? What makes you cry?
- Who loves you?
- What things are you really good at?
- Tell me about a time you felt lonely. How often do you feel lonely?

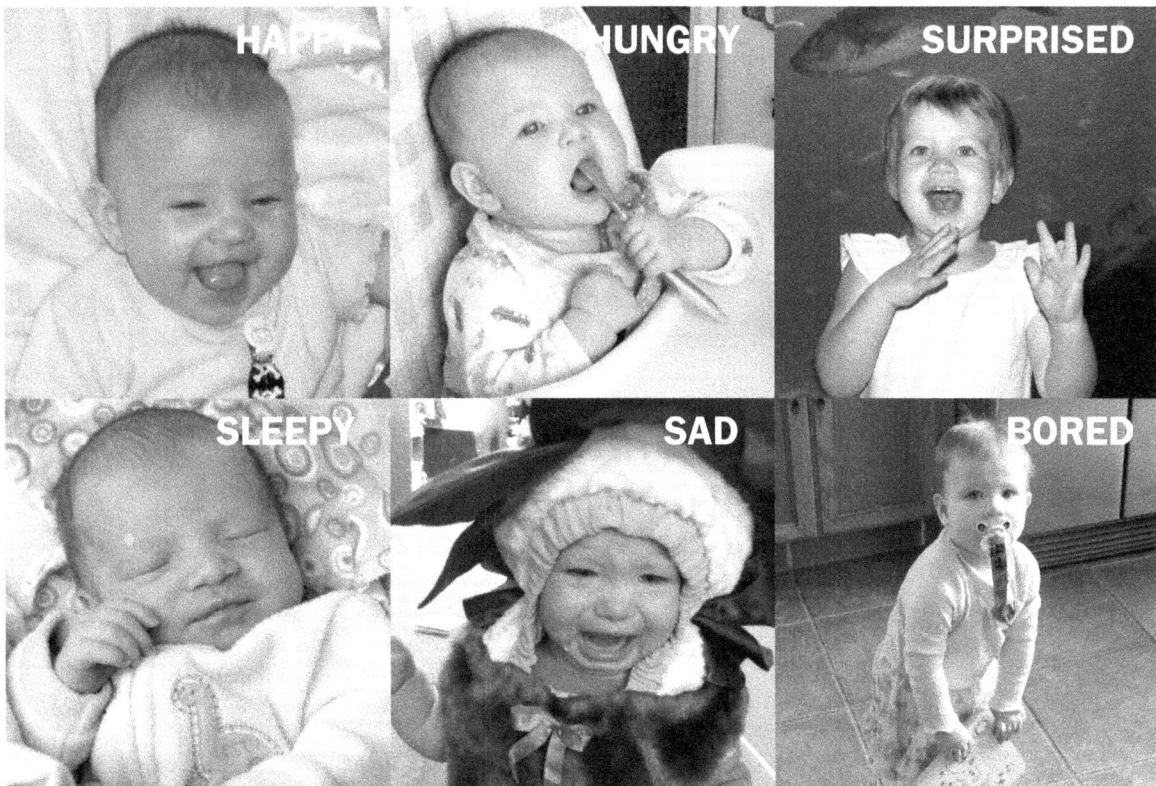

**Photo 4.2:** How Do I Feel? Faces Chart

# CHAPTER GLOSSARY TERMS

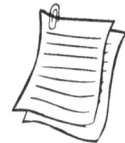

## Mood

**agitation:** Restless, volatile, or erratic emotional behaviour accompanied by a great deal of motor restlessness and often anxiety.

**ambivalent:** The presence of strong, simultaneously contrasting feelings; the ability to hold simultaneously opposite feelings.

**angry:** Strong feelings of annoyance or hostility.

**apathetic:** Feeling no interest.

**apathy:** Lack of interest or emotional involvement in one's surroundings.

**apprehensive:** Mood is characterized by feelings of fear, uncertainty, insecurity, and anxiety; a sense of being threatened. Similar words include anxious, fearful, frightened, high-strung, nervous, overwhelmed, panicked, tense, terrified, and worried.

**blunted:** Diminution of affect; lacking the normal range of responsiveness of mood.

**catastrophic anxiety:** The extreme and overwhelming anxiety felt when a client with an organic brain syndrome becomes aware of the defects in their mentation.

**changeable:** Emotionally labile; frequently changing moods.

**depth:** The level of complexity and extent of feelings and thoughts.

**despair:** Utter abandonment of hope

**duration:** The persistence of the mood, measured in hours, days, weeks, months, or even years.

**dysphoric:** A general feeling of melancholy.

**ecstatic:** Ecstasy; an affect of intense rapture.

**elation:** A high degree of excitement and euphoria in which the client may be expansive, feel invulnerable, and claim that they have never felt better.

**euphoria:** An exaggerated sense of well-being inappropriate to the apparent events.

**euphoric:** A feeling of intense excitement and happiness.

**exultation:** Similar to *euphoria* and *elation* but to a greater degree; intense elation and feelings of grandeur.

**flat:** Similar to *blunted*, indicating an extreme degree of emotional detachment and a lack of normal emotional responsiveness characterized by complete lack of visible emotion and affect.

**grieving:** The alteration in mood or affect that consists of sadness appropriate to a real loss.

**guilt:** Affect associated with self-reproach and the need for punishment.

**insecurity:** Feelings of helplessness and inadequacy in the face of anxiety about one's place, future, and goals.

**labile:** Changeable, unstable.

**melancholic:** Specific type of depressed affect characterized by insomnia and agitation, and sometimes paranoid ideas.

**panic:** An acute, intensive attack of anxiety associated with personality disorganization.

**reactivity:** Whether or not one's mood changes in response to external events or circumstances.

**stability:** The consistency of mood, particularly within the course of a day.

**tearfulness:** Weepiness; moved to tears.

## Affect

**animated:** Facial expression is suitably responsive to the present stimulus or situation. This includes positive responses such as smiling, brightness, and spontaneity.

**appropriate:** Suitable for the ensuing and present activity or environment.

**change pattern:** The rate of change of emotional expression. It is characterized as stable (normal rate of change) or labile (rapid change in emotional expression without external stimuli).

**congruent:** Appropriate response or expression to the presence of stimuli or situation.

**expressionless:** Face registers no specific emotion; appears blank, immobile, unresponsive, and emotionless.

**fatigued:** Face may be haggard or drawn, showing signs of stress, tension, exhaustion, tiredness, and defeat.

**fearful:** Expression reflecting apprehension, fright, tension, or strain.

**grimacing:** Expression consisting of voluntary or involuntary frowning, scowling, or contorted facial movements reflecting disgust, disapproval, and so on.

**incongruent:** Inappropriate response or expression to the presence of stimuli or situation.

**intensity:** The strength of emotional expression. It is characterized as average, flat (complete lack of emotional expression), or blunted (reduced intensity of emotional expression).

**range:** The variation in emotional expression observed throughout the interview. It is characterized as full (normal variation in emotional expression) or constricted (limited variation in emotional expression).

**sad:** Appears melancholic, depressed; reflecting misery, grief, and unhappiness.

## ACTIVITY: WRITING A FOCUSED REVIEW

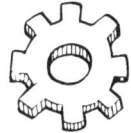

Emotional expression occurs all around us. In movies and television shows, the actors and actresses express emotions both verbally and non-verbally. As a clinician, you need to become attuned to these expressions. This activity provides an opportunity to observe emotional communication as you write a review of a movie or television show. Take this as an opportunity to watch your favourite movie or television show.

- Watch the movie or show from start to finish.
- Take notes while you are watching. You need to note how the characters described their feelings and emotions.
- When you are finished watching, write a brief introduction to summarize the plot or give a synopsis of the storyline. Give a little background of the story, write about the characters and genre of the film or show, and indicate the time and location where the story took place.
- Now focus on one character.
  - How did this character describe their mood?
  - What words did they use?
  - Did what this character say match their behaviour(s)?
- How did you react to this character?
  - How would you describe this character's affect?
  - Was this character able to express a range of emotions?
  - How intense were the emotional expressions?
  - Were the expressions of emotions appropriate for the cultural and social setting?
  - How stable were the emotions? Did the character convey the same emotions consistently throughout the movie or program?
  - Think about the age of the character. How does their expression of emotion correlate with their age?

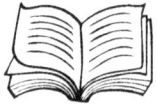

# STUDY QUESTIONS

**1.** What are the five different assessment areas within mood?

_____
_____
_____
_____

**2.** How is affect different than mood? Why is it important to distinguish between the two?

_____
_____
_____
_____
_____

**3.** What are the four different assessment areas within affect?

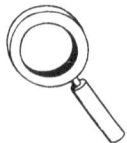

_____
_____
_____
_____

# CASE STUDY

Jaxxon is a heavy-duty equipment operator. He has come to the mental health clinic at the insistence of his wife because she finds him increasingly irritable and has threatened to leave if he doesn't see someone. Over the past couple of months, Jaxxon has felt unusually tired and has had increasingly greater difficulty concentrating at work. Although he has frequent disagreements at work, he is not worried about losing his job; however, he has started to eat lunch alone because there are so many annoying people that he just doesn't want to deal with. This is very different than his usual jovial disposition. During the interview, Jaxxon sits with his hands folded in his lap, eyes cast downward, and has a low monotone voice. He answers questions that are asked of him, but takes one to two minutes before he responds. When asked how he would describe his mood, he responds by saying, "What mood? I feel nothing." When asked what that means, he says, "I just feel numb. I have felt numb for the last month."

## Case Study Questions

1. Describe Jaxxon's affect. Include information on the range, change pattern, intensity, and appropriateness.

   _____

   _____

   _____

   _____

   _____

   _____

   _____

   _____

2. Describe Jaxxon's mood. Include information on the depth, intensity, duration, reactivity, and stability.

   _____

   _____

   _____

   _____

   _____

   _____

   _____

   _____

# CHAPTER 5

## Speech

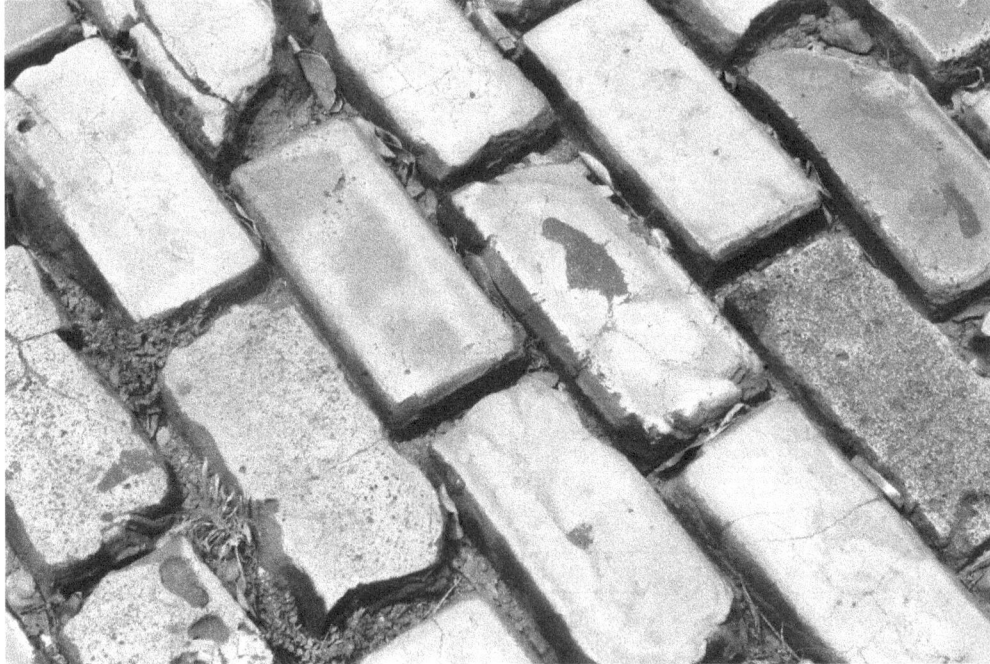

**Photo 5.1:** Used Often but Seldom Seen

Everyone has their own ways of expression. I believe we all have a lot to say,
but finding ways to say it is more than half the battle.
 —*Criss Jami*

## LEARNING OBJECTIVES

**At the completion of this chapter, the reader will be able to:**

- identify the major categories within the speech component of the psychiatric
  mental status examination
- describe assessment indicators for volume, rate, quality, clarity, and
  comprehension

- document objective and subjective assessment findings
- define key terms that may be used in this section of the psychiatric mental status examination
- identify how culture and age affect the assessment of speech

## HOW IS SPEECH ASSESSED?

This section assesses how a person expresses themselves verbally, the physical characteristics and style of their utterances, and how they respond to the clinician's speech. This is also referred to as expressive and receptive language abilities. The mental status exam focuses on what the client is saying and if the clinician understands what the client is saying during the interview. This portion of the mental status examination does not focus on whether or not what the person is saying makes sense or is reasonable. There are many tests that can fully assess expressive and receptive language abilities, but the mental status examination is not one of them. As stated previously, the mental status examination is only a snapshot of *what* is happening—it does not explain *why* things are happening.

There are five primary areas to assess that are related to speech: volume, rate, quality, clarity, and comprehension. Each area has at least one subcomponent. Figure 5.1 outlines these areas in more detail.

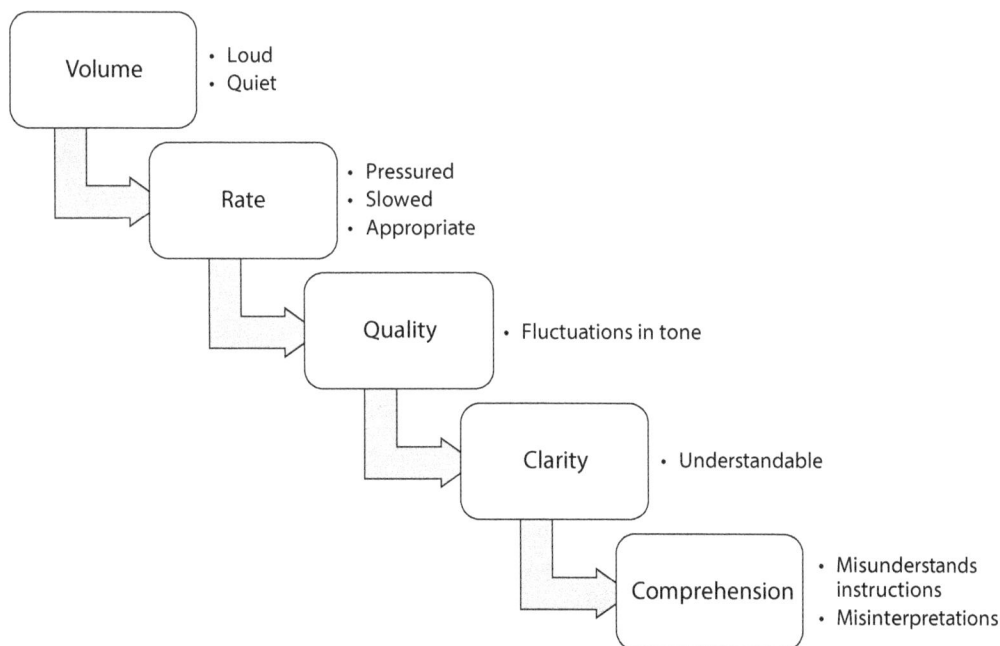

**Figure 5.1:** The Components of Speech

The assessment is conducted while the clinician is engaged in conversation with the client. During your conversation with a client, ask yourself the following questions:

- Does the person say a lot or a little, and do they talk spontaneously or only answer specific questions?
- How fast does the client talk?
- Does the client speak coherently?
- Are there long silences during the conversation?
- Does the person use strange words or grammar, or answer questions in rhymes and puns?
- Do I understand what the person is trying to say?

Evaluation of speech and language can provide important clues to an individual's physical and mental state, thought processes, cognitive organization, and intellectual capacity.

A beginning clinician will often ask, "How do I assess if the client misunderstands instructions or misinterprets something that is said?" This assessment starts soon after meeting the client. For example, if you meet the client in the waiting room and say, "Follow me," but they continue to sit and look directly at you, there may be a misunderstanding. Further assessment will be needed.

If the client's speech is abnormal, a direct quotation illustrating the abnormality should be documented. Abnormality is determined only after the person's age, education, language, and culture have been considered. Box 5.1 provides two examples of documentation in the speech section of the mental status examination.

## BOX 5.1: DOCUMENTING SPEECH FINDINGS

### Ernst

Ernst spoke softly. His speech was clear, coherent, and easy to understand. There were no misinterpretations and he understood all instructions.

### Summer

Summer had a very loud, pressured speech, which made her difficult to understand. She was unable to complete the intake form without the instructions being repeated multiple times, despite her assurances that she understood how to complete the form. When asked about the last time she felt happy, she responded by singing, "Happy is as happy does when happy is happy!"

## SPECIAL CONSIDERATIONS

Speech can be impacted by several factors. If the client has aphasia, this should be noted in this section. When the client's first language is not used during the interview, the clinician should document which language was used. When there are language barriers between the client and the clinician, an interpreter should be used during the interview. When an interpreter is used, the clinician should ask the interpreter about the characteristics of speech demonstrated by the client. The interpreter is asked to base their feedback on normal physical characteristics of speech. Speech differences can also result from a variation in dialects; this is a reflection of shared regional, social, cultural, or ethnic factors. This variation should not be considered an abnormal finding. Knowledge of developmental milestones related to speech should also be used when determining if findings are expected, unexpected, or a common variation.

## CHAPTER GLOSSARY TERMS

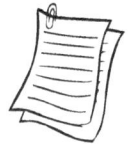

**abusive:** Language that is extremely derogatory.

**accelerated:** Tempo of speech is rapid, giving the impression that a client feels hurried and pushed.

**circumstantial:** Talking around the point but never getting to it.

**clang speech:** Improper use of words based on the sound of the words; similar to punning and rhyming, which is music-like speech.

**clarity:** Describes whether speech is understandable or if there is slurring, mumbling, or stuttering.

**clear:** Speech that follows an orderly, grammatical pattern; words are appropriately used and easily understood.

**emotional:** Speech that is heavily covered with affective tone.

**hesitant:** Speech that is characterized by large pauses between words, as if indicating uncertainty.

**loud:** Greater volume than usual.

**monotone:** Lack of normal modulation in tone.

**mumbled:** Imprecise pronunciation.

**pressured:** Quality of speech; drivenness of the speech.

**quality:** Verbal and non-verbal fluctuations in tone.

**rambling:** A tendency to drift or wander from a subject.

**rate:** The speed of speech, which is further characterized as pressured (very rapid and difficult to interrupt), slowed, or appropriate.

**repetitive:** Repetition of words or phrases.

**slowed:** Enunciation of words is prolonged or pauses between words are increased.

**volume:** Power of sound; it is especially important to comment if the volume of speech is unusually loud or hushed.

**whining:** Speech and tone are fretful, self-pitying, and complaintive.

**whispered:** Soft, breathy voice.

# ACTIVITY: SPEECH LINKAGE WITH OTHER AREAS OF THE MENTAL STATUS EXAMINATION

This activity is provided as a reminder that any one section of the mental status cannot be interpreted in isolation. Information from all sections needs to be used as a whole to produce an accurate assessment.

**Table 5.1:** Speech Linkage with Other Areas of the Mental Status Examination

| Instructions: Indicate whether the following statements are true or false. | TRUE | FALSE |
|---|---|---|
| Speech is an important part of language development. | | |
| It is normal for a child of two years of age to say fewer than 50 words and to not use any two-word combinations (e.g., "more drink," "Mommy gone," "truck go"). | | |
| Difficulty answering questions may be related to biological factors. | | |
| Difficulty sequencing words in sentences is related to speech development. | | |
| An expressive language delay results in difficulty getting across ideas and thoughts. | | |
| A receptive language delay results in difficulty understanding instructions and questions. | | |

| | | |
|---|---|---|
| Language difficulties can result in trouble interacting with peers. | | |
| Language difficulties can result in poor working memory. | | |
| Language difficulties can result in poor attention and concentration. | | |
| Fun play-based activities or games can be used to help motivate a child to learn. | | |

# STUDY QUESTIONS

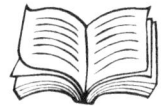

**1.** How do you define rate of speech?

_____

_____

_____

**2.** What are the two types of language skills that are assessed in the speech component of the mental status exam?

_____

_____

_____

_____

**3.** What types of medical conditions might affect a person's speech? Refer to chapter 1 for ideas.

_____

_____

_____

_____

_____

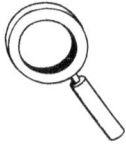

# CASE STUDY

Kaseem is eight years old. His mother tells you that Kaseem is getting in trouble at school. He is fighting with other children. The teacher has told her that Kaseem is having difficulty verbally expressing his thoughts and seems to get frustrated easily. Kaseem's teacher tells his mother that she doesn't understand what is happening. Kaseem is a quiet boy who doesn't talk much. He has never had many friends and has always seemed to prefer to be alone. When the clinician meets Kaseem, they start to talk about his favourite things to do. Kaseem thinks for a while and then says, "Lego." When asked what he last built, after another long pause, he replies, "Car building yesterday." During the interview, Kaseem's sentences don't always make sense. He leaves out key words and often confuses verb tense.

## Case Study Questions

Using the information presented in the above case study, answer the following questions.

1.  Is there information that describes the volume of Kaseem's speech for the purposes of the mental status exam?

    _____
    _____
    _____

2.  What information is described in relation to rate of speaking?

    _____
    _____
    _____
    _____

3.  Is there information that can be used to determine how clarity of speech was assessed?

    _____
    _____
    _____
    _____

**4.** Is there information that describes the clarity of Kaseem's speech for the purposes of the mental status exam?

_____

_____

_____

_____

**5.** What information is described related to Kaseem's level of comprehension?

_____

_____

_____

_____

_____

# CHAPTER 6

## Thought Processes

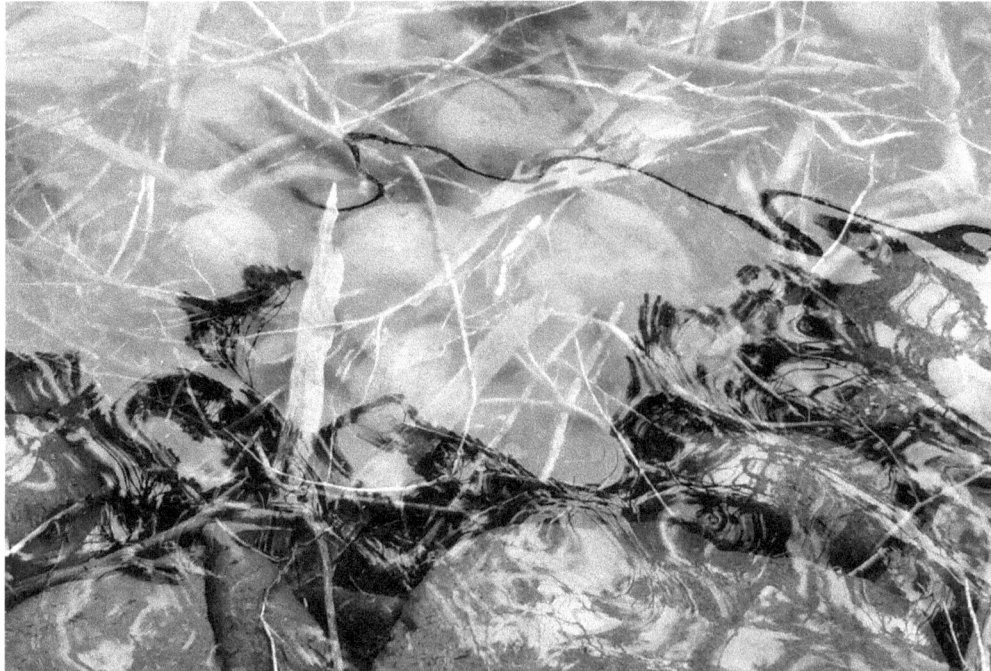

**Photo 6.1:** To Understand Thought Processes, We Must Look Under the Surface

The world as we have created it is a process of our thinking. It cannot be changed without changing our thinking.
   —*Albert Einstein*

## LEARNING OBJECTIVES

**At the completion of this chapter, the reader will be able to:**

- identify the major categories within the thought processes component of the psychiatric mental status examination
- describe assessment indicators for rate of thought, flow of ideas, and form of thought

- document objective and subjective assessment findings
- define key terms that may be used in this section of the psychiatric mental status examination
- identify how age affects the assessment of thought processes

# HOW ARE THOUGHT PROCESSES ASSESSED?

The relationship between thought process and speech is unclear; however, in practical terms, comprehensive assessment of thought process is dependent upon intact speech and language comprehension abilities. In this section of the psychiatric mental status examination, the clinician describes the way in which the client's thinking flows from topic to topic as observed during the interview. Basically, the clinician is documenting the way a person thinks. There are three primary components to this assessment: rate of thought, flow of ideas, and form of thought.

How can these components be assessed? Each clinician, over time, will develop questions that work well for them and the people they normally assess. Below are a few sample questions that will help as you begin to develop your confidence in assessing thought processes.

## Rate of Thought

Does the client appear to think rapidly or slowly? Do they show a paucity of ideas or an overabundance of ideas? When documenting findings in this area, the clinician may describe the rate of thought as rapid or slow, or they may note that the client has an overabundance of ideas.

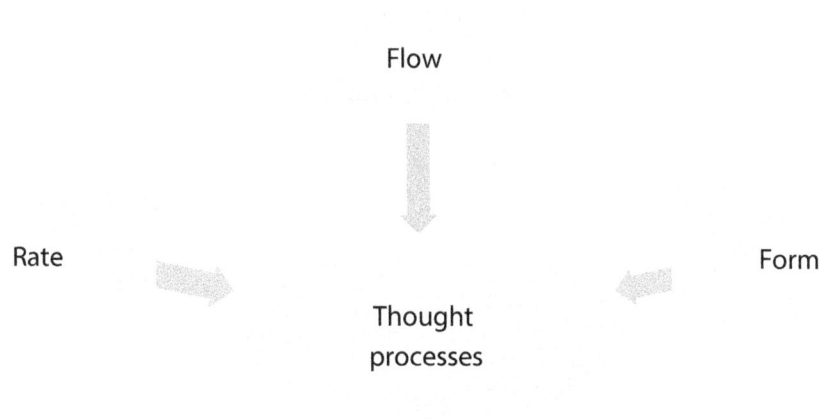

**Figure 6.1:** Components of Thought Processes

## Flow of Ideas

When assessing the flow of ideas, the clinician will ask themself the following questions: Is there a connectedness or organization to the person's thoughts? Are the connections logical and easily understood? Are they relevant or irrelevant, coherent or incoherent? There are several terms that can be used when documenting flow of ideas, including the following:

- tangentially
- circumstantiality
- flight of ideas
- loosening of associations
- echolalia
- word salad
- neologisms
- perseveration

## Form of Thought

Form of thought relates to how coherent, logical, and goal-directed the ideas presented by the client are. There are many questions the clinician can ask themself to assess this area when they reflect on the content of the interview, including the following: Does the person seem to be preoccupied or hesitant, or do their thoughts seem to be blocked? Is the person able to think beyond the most overt meaning? Is their thinking "black and white"? Do the answers given actually answer the questions asked? Does the person provide very little detail or do they provide an excessive amount of irrelevant detail when responding to questions? When completing the documentation about their findings in this area of the mental status exam, the clinician may use terms and phrases such as thought blocking, paucity of ideas, impoverished, overly inclusive, or non-sequiturious. Box 6.1 provides two examples of thought process documentation.

## BOX 6.1: DOCUMENTING THOUGHT PROCESS FINDINGS

### Georgia
Her thought processes were of average speed, logical, and congruent with the conversation.

### Dahlia
Dahlia had an overabundance of ideas. Each idea was loosely connected to the previous idea. Generally, there was a loosening of associations; however, there

were several times during the interview when the connections between ideas were incoherent, yet she provided an exorbitant amount of detail.

## SPECIAL CONSIDERATIONS

Due to the complex relationship between speech and thought processes, it is imperative that an interpreter be used to support the client and the clinician when they are unable to verbally communicate with one another. When interviewing children and adolescents, it is important to consider age-appropriate development as the baseline for assessment.

## CHAPTER GLOSSARY TERMS

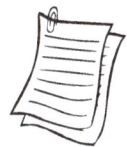

**blocking:** Intellectual processes that are characterized by sudden stoppages in the sequential flow of thought and speech.

**flight of ideas:** Thought patterns consisting of a rapid succession of ideas with little or no visible connection; a tendency for the client to start talking about one subject, then rapidly switch to another subject, then another, with little connection between topics.

**illogical:** Speech that lacks coherence, is disorganized and unintelligible, and may consist of words and phrases that are garbled, vague, and nonsensical, including neologisms and word salad. The speech pattern may be broken down by irregular interruptions, halting, and blocking.

**irrelevant:** Thoughts appear to be out of place and not normally associated with the topic at hand.

**logical:** Speech follows an orderly grammatical pattern, and is appropriately used and easy to understand.

**poverty (paucity) of ideas:** Absence or scarcity of thoughts or imagination.

**preoccupation:** A state of daydreaming; the client appears to be out of touch with their surroundings and absorbed in their own thoughts.

**relevant:** Related to the topic.

**tangential thinking:** A disturbance in thinking in which the client is unable to express their ideas because they digress or are derailed; they never quite get to the point.

**thought flow:** The organization or "connectedness" of thinking. It is characterized as logical when there are clear and easily understood connections between thoughts, and as disjointed when these connections are unclear and difficult to follow.

**thought form:** The way (form) in which thoughts are expressed. It is characterized as concrete (inability to think beyond the most overt meaning), impoverished (little meaningful information contained in the conversation), or overly inclusive (excessive, irrelevant detail).

**thought rate:** May be revealed through direct questioning or inferred based on the rate of speech. It is characterized as rapid, slowed, or appropriate.

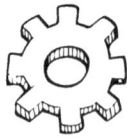

# ACTIVITY: ALPHABET SOUP PUZZLE

Figuring out how a person thinks is often a challenge. There are many factors that affect thought processes, ranging from developmental stage to speech, from physical injury to illness. The following activity provides an opportunity to filter through distractors as you find the embedded words.

There is one place for each letter of the alphabet in 26 empty squares in table 6.1. Fill in each letter so that a word of at least five letters is formed, reading across only. Not all of the letters to the left and right of the empty box will be used. It is up to you to discover which letters are needed to complete familiar words. Some letters may fit in more than one of the empty squares to complete words; however, only one arrangement of all the letters of the alphabet will complete a word in each row. For example, in the first row, inserting a *U* completes the word *hallucinated*. Fill in the rest of the empty spaces to create words related to the mental status examination. When you have filled in all of the blank boxes, all of the letters of the alphabet will have been used. Plurals and proper names are not allowed.

**Table 6.1:** Alphabet Soup Puzzle

| | | | | | | | | | | | | | | | |
|---|---|---|---|---|---|---|---|---|---|---|---|---|---|---|---|
| A | A | N | C | H | A | L | L | U | | C | I | N | A | T | E | D |
| B | D | O | R | G | A | N | I | | E | D | E | F | E | N | S |
| C | E | C | H | O | P | E | U | | H | O | B | I | A | L | S |
| D | L | S | I | O | D | R | A | | A | T | I | C | O | M | P |
| E | M | I | S | I | D | E | N | | P | A | T | H | Y | P | O |
| F | S | A | R | C | A | G | I | | A | T | E | D | E | N | T |
| G | Q | U | E | S | T | I | N | | U | I | R | E | L | I | T |
| H | D | I | F | F | P | L | A | | E | C | H | P | R | A | X |
| I | P | O | S | T | U | R | I | | Y | S | T | O | N | I | C |
| J | U | P | E | R | P | L | E | | E | D | R | O | W | S | Y |
| K | O | V | E | R | A | B | U | | I | T | H | D | R | A | W |
| L | N | O | N | J | U | B | E | | A | V | I | O | U | R | A |
| M | R | E | L | A | T | I | H | | P | E | R | O | N | S | H |
| N | L | I | N | C | O | N | G | | U | E | N | T | I | O | N |
| O | M | I | S | I | D | E | N | | B | S | E | S | S | E | T |
| P | D | E | M | E | N | D | E | | I | R | I | U | M | U | S |
| Q | G | R | A | N | D | I | O | | E | G | L | E | C | T | Y |
| R | U | N | L | A | B | I | L | | Q | U | E | S | T | I | O |
| S | R | E | F | E | R | E | N | | U | D | G | M | E | N | T |
| T | D | I | S | F | R | A | N | | E | G | L | E | C | T | E |
| U | F | L | U | R | T | A | T | | L | L | U | S | I | O | N |
| V | I | N | S | I | F | I | D | | E | T | F | U | L | L | Y |
| W | C | H | A | F | E | A | R | | U | L | I | Z | A | T | E |
| X | E | X | P | R | E | D | E | | P | A | I | R | I | O | N |
| Y | P | H | A | G | I | A | E | | A | S | I | V | E | U | N |
| Z | D | I | S | A | R | A | M | | I | V | A | L | E | N | T |

## STUDY QUESTIONS

1. What are the three components of a thought process assessment and what do each of them mean?

_____
_____
_____
_____
_____
_____
_____
_____
_____
_____
_____
_____
_____
_____

2. Describe the relationship between speech and thought processes.

_____
_____
_____
_____

3. When a client displays speech abnormalities, what strategies can be used to facilitate communication so thought processes can be assessed?

_____
_____
_____
_____
_____

## CASE STUDY

Dahlia is an eight-year-old with an overabundance of ideas. She speaks rapidly and jumps from topic to topic. She has some trouble pronouncing her "z" and "th" sounds; however, she was generally understood during the interview. Each idea was loosely connected to the previous idea. Generally, there was a loosening of associations. She began talking about princesses, then immediately went to horses, bunnies, Easter egg hunts, and Santa Claus, and then asked why Santa Claus didn't give her a birthday present. Several times during the interview the connections between ideas were less coherent, yet she provided an exorbitant amount of detail with every description. Three months ago, Dahlia was riding her bicycle without a helmet and hit a tree. Since that time, she has demonstrated periods of excitement with pressure of speech alternating with periods of extreme fatigue. Dahlia also complains about headaches.

## Case Study Questions

Complete table 6.2 to compare expected findings to expected variations and unexpected findings in Dahlia's case.

**Table 6.2:** Thought Process Variations

| Assessment area | Expected findings | Expected variations | Unexpected findings/ further assessment required |
|---|---|---|---|
| *Rate of thought* | | | |
| *Flow of Ideas* | | | |
| *Form of thought* | | | |

# CHAPTER 7

## Thought Content

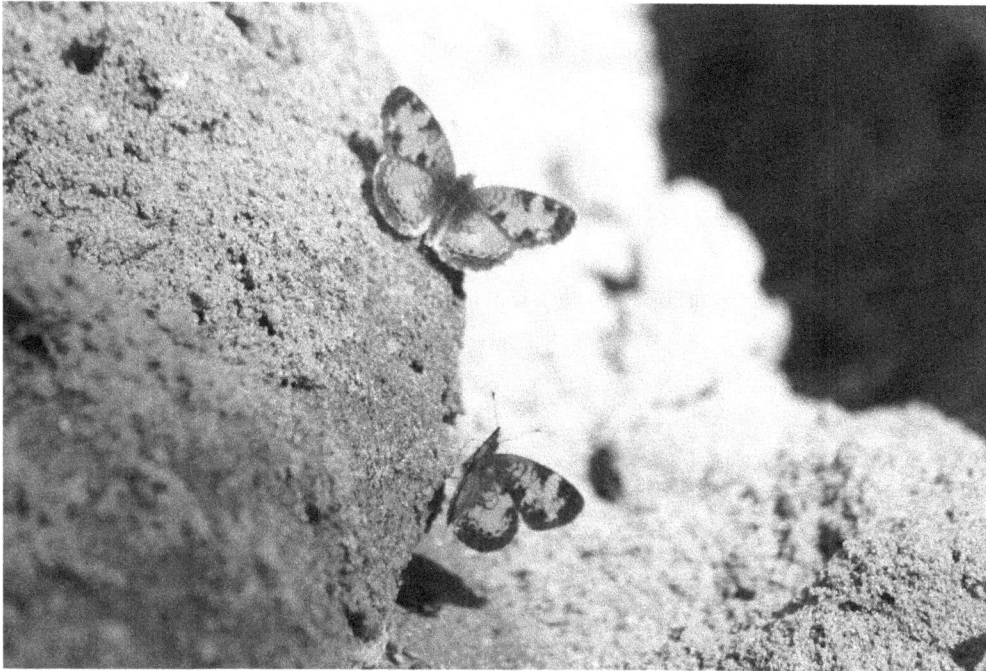

**Photo 7.1:** I Think about Flying—What Do You Think about?

You are only as free as you think you are and freedom will always be as real as you believe it to be.
—*Robert M. Drake*

## LEARNING OBJECTIVES

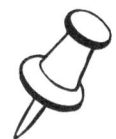

**At the completion of this chapter, the reader will be able to:**

- identify the major categories within the thought content component of the psychiatric mental status examination
- describe assessment indicators for thought content

- · document objective and subjective assessment findings
- · define key terms that may be used in this section of the psychiatric mental status examination
- · identify how culture and age affect the assessment of thought content

## HOW IS THOUGHT CONTENT ASSESSED?

In this area of the mental status examination, the client's present thoughts and preoccupations are described. Some clinicians will ask their clients what they see as their main worries, and if they have anxieties or preoccupations with their present situation, the future, or the past, or with their own safety or the safety of others. Thoughts about harming oneself or others are extremely important to assess. Due to the importance of understanding the current level of risk that results from suicidal or homicidal ideation, chapter 8 focuses solely on completing a risk assessment. The remainder of this chapter covers thought disturbances that do not pose an immediate and imminent danger to oneself or others.

The goal of this chapter is to help novice clinicians familiarize themselves with how to assess thought content. When the clinician assesses thought content, they attempt to understand *what* the person thinks about (*how* a person thinks was discussed in detail in chapter 6). Once the clinician understands what their client is thinking about, they then need to make a determination about the "normalcy" of the client's thoughts. When making this determination, clinicians will ask themselves the following questions: Are the thoughts reasonable, based on the person's current experiences? Are the thoughts causing this person distress? Would other people, with similar life experiences, have similar thoughts? Would their thoughts cause them a comparable level of distress?

Answers to these questions provide the clinician with clues to determine if there is an underlying thought disorder. Findings in this area provide information related to a number of symptoms, outlined in box 7.1; however, it is important to remember that the mental status exam is about reporting presenting symptoms. It is a snapshot. Because pathology in thought content is present in many psychiatric disorders, clinicians will often start to formulate potential diagnoses, which will help guide treatment decisions. For example, a person may believe that they are starting to rot from the inside, as they believe the sensations they feel are a result of their internal organs dying; however, it is essential to guard against using only one part of the mental status examination to formulate a diagnosis. This section of the mental status exam must be considered along with all of the other parts of the exam, in addition to a full biopsychosocial and spiritual assessment in order to make a responsible diagnosis.

## BOX 7.1: EXAMPLES OF THOUGHT DISORDER SYMPTOMS

- anti-social urges
- compulsions
- delusions
- ideas of influence
- ideas of reference
- magical thinking
- obsessions
- overvalued ideas
- paranoia
- phobias
- physical concerns
- preoccupations
- ruminations
- suspiciousness
- thought broadcasting
- thought insertion
- thought withdrawal

Changes in thought content can result in altered beliefs (delusions), behaviours (compulsions), attitudes (ideas of reference), and values (ideas of influence). People who experience depression, addiction, and dementia and people who are guarded, suspicious, or otherwise odd during the interview have a higher probability of experiencing abnormalities in thought content.

When assessing for delusional content, specific questions must be included in the interview. For example, during an interview with a person who reports feeling depressed, the clinician could say, "Sometimes depression causes people to have unusual experiences, like feeling that others are trying to harm them. Has that happened to you?" A person who is seeking assistance with symptoms related to an addiction might be asked, "Have drugs ever caused your mind to play tricks on you? Do you feel as though someone is with you when they are not or are you having paranoid ideas?" When interviewing a person who has dementia, the clinician could ask, "When you misplace things, do you sometimes think that they've been stolen?" or "Have you heard or seen people coming into your house?" If the person is suspicious, the clinician could ask, "Have people been harassing you or trying to harm you?" Once the person answers these types of questions, further assessment is needed to determine if their beliefs are grounded in reality or if they are in fact delusions.

Documentation in this area should describe a person's fears, worries, and anxieties. Attention should be paid to whether the anxieties are generalized and non-specific (free-floating), or specifically related to particular situations, activities, persons, or objects (phobias). When describing anxiety, there can be an overlap between emotional state and thought content. The physical observations previously made that indicate an anxious state, such as moist hands; perspiring forehead; tense, rigid posture; sitting on the edge of the seat; motor restlessness; a strained or quavering voice; hand wringing; or fidgeting with one's fingers or clothing, should be re-emphasized. Box 7.2 provides two examples of thought content descriptions.

## BOX 7.2: DOCUMENTING THOUGHT CONTENT FINDINGS

### Bilan

Thought content focused primarily around her worries regarding money, her relationships, and low self-esteem.

### Amar

Amar has begun to isolate himself from other people. He describes others as trying to put thoughts into his head. He no longer watches television as he believes a local news broadcaster can read his mind. He describes having panic attacks that are often worse late at night. He tries to deal with them by making himself numb and not feeling anything; however, he reports that this makes him particularly vulnerable to the neighbours reading his mind.

## SPECIAL CONSIDERATIONS

The normality of thought content needs to be assessed based on the client's cultural context and social system. If the client's belief system differs from the clinician's, this does not mean that the client is delusional. Further assessment is required for the clinician to understand what is happening from the perspective of their client. It is essential that clinicians have well-developed cultural sensitivities in order to make an accurate assessment.

In addition, knowledge of normal growth and development is critical to accurately assess this area of the mental status exam. For example, young children may report hearing Santa Claus on the roof of their home on Christmas Eve. This is a demonstration of magical thinking that is age appropriate; therefore, this alone is not indicative of a thought disturbance.

# CHAPTER GLOSSARY TERMS

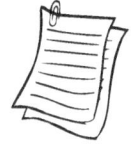

**compulsions:** Involuntary, uncontrollable, repetitive behavioural acts or rituals that the client feels compelled to carry out because of a feeling of anxiety.

**delusions:** Beliefs that are not true to fact, cannot be corrected by an appeal to reason of the individual, and are out of harmony with their educational and cultural background.

**delusions of control:** False beliefs that one is being manipulated by others.

**delusions of grandeur:** False beliefs consisting of an exaggerated concept of one's own importance.

**delusions of infidelity:** False beliefs that one's lover is unfaithful.

**delusions of reference:** False beliefs that the behaviour of others refers to oneself.

**delusions of self-accusation:** False feelings of remorse or guilt.

**hypochondriacal thoughts:** Occur when a client is morbidly concerned about their physical health or persistently complains of various physical ailments, though medical evidence will not support their claim.

**ideas of influence:** Feelings that one is capable of influencing the behaviour of others or situations through one's thoughts or desires; closely related to grandiose delusions.

**ideas of reference:** Misinterpretation of incidents and events in the outside world as having a direct, personal significance, or reference to oneself.

**obsessions:** Thoughts, feelings, or ideas that intrude upon a person's conscious awareness, and are accompanied by an effort to resist this intrusion and an awareness that these thoughts are abnormal.

**persecutory delusions:** Over-suspiciousness leading to false persecutory ideas or beliefs.

**phobias:** Irrational fear of an object or situation usually accompanied by behaviour to avoid that object or situation. In a phobia, the client retains the knowledge that their fear is unrealistic.

# ACTIVITY: DEVELOPMENTAL REFRESHER

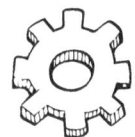

When evaluating thought content, it is essential to consider the client's developmental stage. The following activity provides an opportunity to recall normal developmental tasks. Fill in the information missing from table 7.1.

**Table 7.1:** Developmental Refresher

| Age | Erikson | Piaget | Developmental tasks | Coping skills |
|---|---|---|---|---|
| **Infancy (0–1 year)** | Basic trust versus mistrust | Sensorimotor (birth–2 years) | | |

*continued*

| Age | Erikson | Piaget | Developmental tasks | Coping skills |
|---|---|---|---|---|
| *Early childhood (2–3 years)* | Autonomy versus shame | Preoperational (2–7 years) | | |
| *Play age (4–5 years)* | Initiative versus guilt | Preoperational (2–7 years) | | |
| *School age (6–11 years)* | Industry versus inferiority | Concrete operational (7–11 years) | | |
| *Adolescence (12–19 years)* | Identity versus confusion | Formal operational (adolescent to adult) | | |
| *Early adulthood (20–25 years)* | Intimacy versus isolation | Formal operational (adolescent to adult) | | |
| *Adulthood (26–64 years)* | Generativity versus stagnation | Formal operational (adolescent to adult) | | |

| Age | Erikson | Piaget | Developmental tasks | Coping skills |
|---|---|---|---|---|
| **Old age (65 years to death)** | Integrity versus despair | Formal operational (adolescent to adult) | | |

# STUDY QUESTIONS

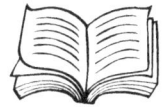

**1.** What is a phobia?

_____

_____

_____

**2.** Why is a phobia considered abnormal thought content?

_____

_____

_____

**3.** How does a clinician determine if thought content is abnormal?

_____

_____

_____

_____

# CASE STUDY

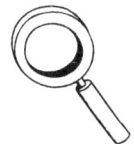

James is a 24-year-old male who lives at home with his parents. He works in the mailroom of his uncle's law firm. He has had this job for the last four years. His elderly parents drive him to work every day as he is worried that his actions have caused, or will cause, harm to others. He has never driven a vehicle as he is sure that this will result in someone's death. Because of his belief that he will be responsible for harming another, he constantly re-checks everything he does to make sure that no one is hurt. He has been able to maintain his job because his primary responsibility is to sort the mail. He does not deliver the mail around the office. His mother walks with him to the mailroom when they arrive at the office, he eats his lunch in the mailroom, and at the end of the day his father picks him up from the mailroom. James has intrusive thoughts that are having a significant impact on his ability to process any external information. Over the last month, James's hygiene has been deteriorating as his thoughts have impacted his ability to get ready for work. His intrusive thoughts decrease when he repeats tasks—but he must repeat them at least three times for this to be effective. The other person who works in the mailroom and delivers the mail has always thought that James was strange, but that it was just his personality. Now his co-worker is starting to complain because of his body odour. James reports that this is "stressing him out."

## Case Study Activity: What Is Expected versus Unexpected?

Based on the case study above, use table 7.2 to identify what variations in thought content are present, when these symptoms could be expected, and when these symptoms may be an acceptable variation that would not prompt further investigation.

**Table 7.2:** Thought Content Variation Table

| Circle which of the listed symptoms are present in the preceding case study. | Identify when these symptoms could be an expected finding. | Identify when these symptoms could be a common variation in clinical presentation. |
|---|---|---|
| *Phobias* | | |
| *Obsessions* | | |
| *Compulsions* | | |

| | | |
|---|---|---|
| *Delusions* | | |
| *Physical concerns* | | |
| *Anti-social urges* | | |
| *Ideas of reference* | | |
| *Ideas of influence* | | |
| *Thought insertion* | | |
| *Thought broadcasting* | | |
| *Thought withdrawal* | | |

# CHAPTER 8

## Risk Assessment

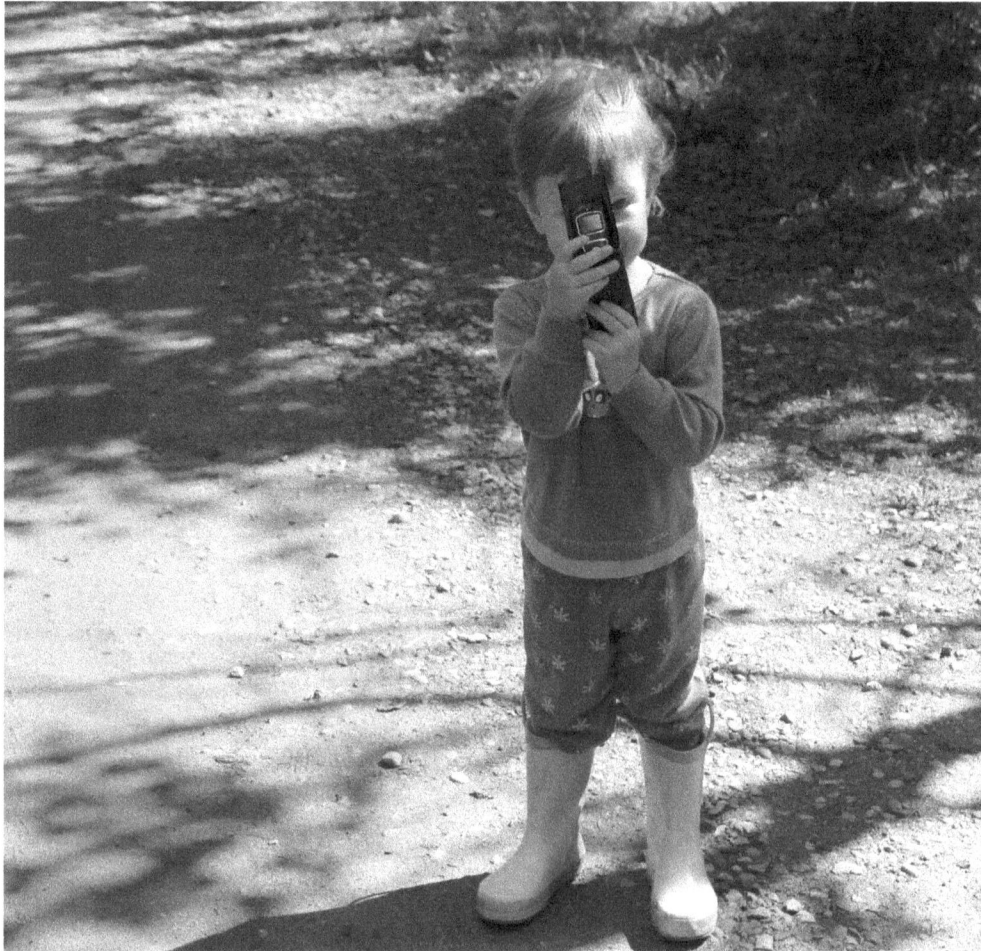

**Photo 8.1:** You Can't Tell by Looking

To be or not to be—that is the question:
Whether 'tis nobler in the mind to suffer
The slings and arrows of outrageous fortune,
Or to take arms against a sea of troubles
And, by opposing, end them?
   —Shakespeare, Hamlet

# LEARNING OBJECTIVES

**At the completion of this chapter, the reader will be able to:**

- identify the components of the psychiatric mental status examination that are related to risk
- describe how to assess each of the following major psychiatric mental status assessment areas: thought content, delusions, persecutory hallucinations, and mood
- document objective and subjective assessment findings
- define key terms that may be used in this section of the psychiatric mental status examination
- identify how age may affect the assessment of risk

# WHAT IS A RISK ASSESSMENT?

During every mental status examination, the clinician will ask the client about suicidal and homicidal thoughts. Each clinician will develop their own routine as to when they ask about these thoughts and potential plans. Most novice clinicians experience discomfort when starting to ask people about this area; however, just as surgical nurses ask their clients about pain, mental health practitioners need to ask their clients about psychological pain that can manifest itself as suicidal ideation when turned inward and homicidal ideation when turned outward. It is important for novice clinicians to keep in mind that a mental status examination is a clinical interaction, rather than a social interaction, and that the mental status examination requires that the interviewer to explore all aspects of thought and mood, regardless of the sensitive nature of the topic. Failure to do so may result in an incomplete or inaccurate risk assessment and impair the ability of the interviewer to effectively intervene.

Just as the overall mental status examination is a snapshot in time, this section is also considered a snapshot. The level of risk is reflective of the current time and place. The level of risk to one's self and others fluctuates over the course of most mental illnesses and, as a result, must be frequently reassessed.

There are four specific areas that must be investigated to determine the current level of risk: thought content, delusions, command hallucinations, and mood. The interviewer must inquire about these specific areas if the client does not mention them. Refer back to chapter 7 for more information about delusions. Hallucinations are briefly discussed in this chapter, though a more detailed discussion can be found in chapter 9. The assessment of mood was discussed in chapter 4.

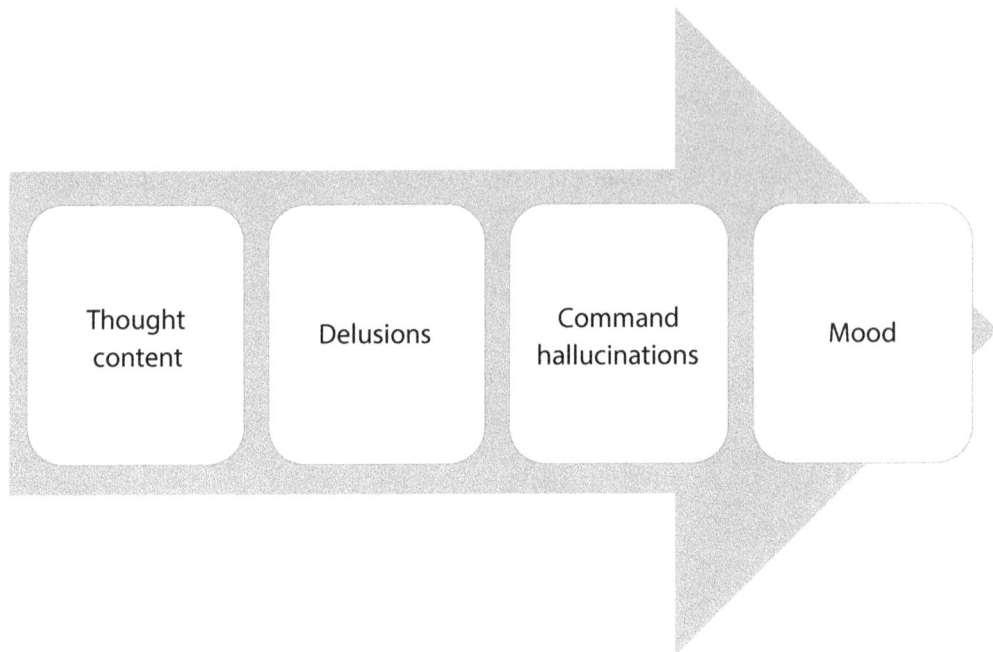

**Figure 8.1:** Essential Assessment Areas

## How Do You Ask about Suicidal or Homicidal Thought Content?

Most professionals who work in mental health develop a set of assessment questions that they use regularly. Depending on the client's cultural needs, the questions may be changed slightly, but the clinician will always assess for suicidal or homicidal ideation. The clinician will first ask, "Have you thought about harming yourself or someone else?" They will then ask, "Have you ever had thoughts about wanting to die?" If the answer to both questions is no, the clinician should let the client know that these questions will be asked several times over the course of their care. They are a required part of mental health assessment. If the answer to either or both questions is yes, further assessment is needed. The following list provides examples of follow-up questions that can be used to obtain more information:

- How long have you had these types of thoughts?
- How often do you have these types of thoughts?
- How intense are these thoughts?
- How persistent are these thoughts?
- Are you able to control these thoughts?
- Do you have the desire to act on these thoughts?
- With having these thoughts, what is your intention?
- Are there times when these thoughts are more intense?

- Are there times when it feels like you are unable to control, or have decreasing control over, these thoughts?
- Would you like help to control or reduce these thoughts?
- Do you have a plan to act on these thoughts?
- Tell me about your plan.

## How Do You Ask about Delusions?

People who are delusional have faith, confidence, acceptance, and conviction that their thoughts and experiences are true; therefore, asking someone if they are delusional is not effective. The type of delusions that increase the risk of harming oneself or another person generally fall into two categories: paranoid and jealous. Occasionally, a somatization delusion may result in the individual experiencing increased hopelessness. These types of thoughts increase a person's psychological pain, which can increase thoughts about wanting to die. The following are examples of questions that will help to identify whether delusional thought content is present:

- What has been on your mind recently?
- Do you find that others disagree with your opinions or views?
- Are you involved in a relationship? How are things going?
- Do you hope to become involved in a relationship?

The answers to these questions alone will not allow the clinician to determine if the thought content is delusional. Follow-up questions are needed to deepen the assessment. The following are examples of follow-up questions:

- How do you know this?
- What do your friends say about this?
- When did this all start?
- How have things worked out so far?

## How Do You Ask about Command Hallucinations?

Determining the content of hallucinations is much easier than assessing if thought content is delusional. When assessing hallucinations, you are asking about what the person hears, sees, tastes, feels, or smells. When assessing for risk, you are assessing for a special type of auditory (something that is heard) hallucination—a command hallucination. This means that you are trying to determine if the person is hearing someone tell them to hurt themself or someone else. First ask the client if they hear someone, or something, telling them to harm themself or someone else. Then, following the same pattern as you would when assessing suicidal or homicidal thoughts, further assessment is needed if the person is experiencing command hallucinations. Here are some potential questions you could ask of an individual who is experiencing command hallucinations:

- How long have you heard these instructions?
- How often do you hear these instructions?
- How persistent are the instructions or the voice providing them?
- Are you able to control what you hear?
- Do you have the desire to act on these instructions?
- As you are being told what you should do, what is your intention? Do you plan to act on these instructions?
- Are there times when these voices are more intense?
- Are there times when it feels like you are unable to control, or have decreasing control over, these voices?
- Would you like help to control, or quiet, these voices?
- What effect is this experience having on your life?

Communicating this information to the health care team is essential. The team members work together to reduce the risk of the client harming themself or others; therefore, the presence or absence of suicidal and homicidal ideation, as well as its severity or urgency, must be specifically documented. Box 8.1 provides examples of documentation for the risk assessment area within the mental status exam.

## BOX 8.1: DOCUMENTING INFORMATION ABOUT RISK

### James
He denies the presence of any thoughts related to harming himself or others. There is no evidence to suggest delusional thought content or command hallucinations.

### Raine
There is some suicidal ideation; however, she does not have a plan nor does she think it's likely that she will harm herself. She denies any thoughts of harming others.

### Martha
Martha has attempted suicide on three occasions. Currently she denies having any suicidal or homicidal ideations. She states that her children need her and she would not consider suicide at this time. The last time she thought about suicide

she thought briefly about taking the kids with her. Martha states that she still feels guilty about even thinking about harming her children; however, she is concerned about her own safety as her ex-husband abused her in the past and is becoming increasingly angry as she has given him an ultimatum about seeing their children. She reports that he will never have custody of the kids.

### Sam

Sam describes deprecating command hallucinations. These include a woman's voice repeatedly telling him that he just doesn't "have what it takes" to kill himself. This voice started about three weeks ago after a breakup with his girlfriend. Since that time, the voice has gotten louder, more frequent, and more difficult to control. It started by saying things like, "Who would ever want to go out with you?" and "She is better off with anyone but you." Sam reports thinking about death before the breakup, but now he thinks about it every day. The intensity of the thoughts is increasing. The voice tells him to "go and shoot himself." He doesn't want to but states, "This [voice] is driving me crazy." He has thought about taking his father's gun and going into the ravine one night and permanently blowing the voice out of his head. On a scale of 1 (no chance of doing this) to 10 (I will do it), Sam rates himself a 6. Information was provided to Sam about emergency mental health crisis lines. He has agreed to call the crisis line and contact his psychiatrist if this rating increases.

# SPECIAL CONSIDERATIONS

At the beginning of the interview, the client should be informed that there are limitations on what the clinician is able to keep confidential. In most jurisdictions, these limitations include reports of significant risk to oneself or others, and if there is a court order to release the files. Establishing trust is a significant step in developing a therapeutic relationship. It is important that clients of all ages, particularly adolescents, are aware that there are situations in which information must be shared with others.

By the time most children reach eight years of age, they will have an understanding of death and suicide; they will also have the capacity to plan and carry out their plans (Soole, Kolves, & De Leo, 2015). The World Health Organization (2014) has identified that death by suicide is the second leading cause of death in 15- to 29-year-olds worldwide. It is therefore as important to explore this subject with children and adolescents as it is with adults. Box 8.2 provides some questions that can be used to begin the assessment of risk with children.

## BOX 8.2: ASKING A CHILD ABOUT SUICIDE

The starting point of all risk assessments is establishing a relationship. Although the following questions will not be the first that are asked when you initially meet with your client, they may be helpful in exploring a person's history with suicide, their engagement with potential support systems, active versus passive ideation, and the presence of changeable risk factors.

- Do you think you have been under a lot of stress lately?
- Have you ever felt like life is not worth living?
- Have you thought about dying?
- Have you thought about your own death?
- Have you wished you could go to sleep and not wake up?
- In the past month, have you felt so bad that you have considered harming or killing yourself?
- What do you think about suicide?
- Is suicide something any of your friends talk about?

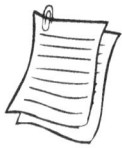

## CHAPTER GLOSSARY TERMS

**homicidal:** Intent to kill another person.
**intensity:** The amount of or strength of thoughts.
**intent:** Level of determination.
**plan:** Decisions regarding method that would be used to harm oneself or another.
**suicidal:** Intent to kill oneself.

## ACTIVITY: RISK ASSESSMENT WORD SEARCH

The following activity is a reminder that any one section of the mental status exam cannot be interpreted in isolation. Information from all sections needs to be considered as a whole to obtain an accurate assessment.

Find the words listed below.

- agitated
- ambivalent
- apathy
- compulsion
- control
- delusions
- despair
- hallucination
- incongruent
- indifferent
- irritable
- judgement
- lonely
- memory
- sleeping
- volition

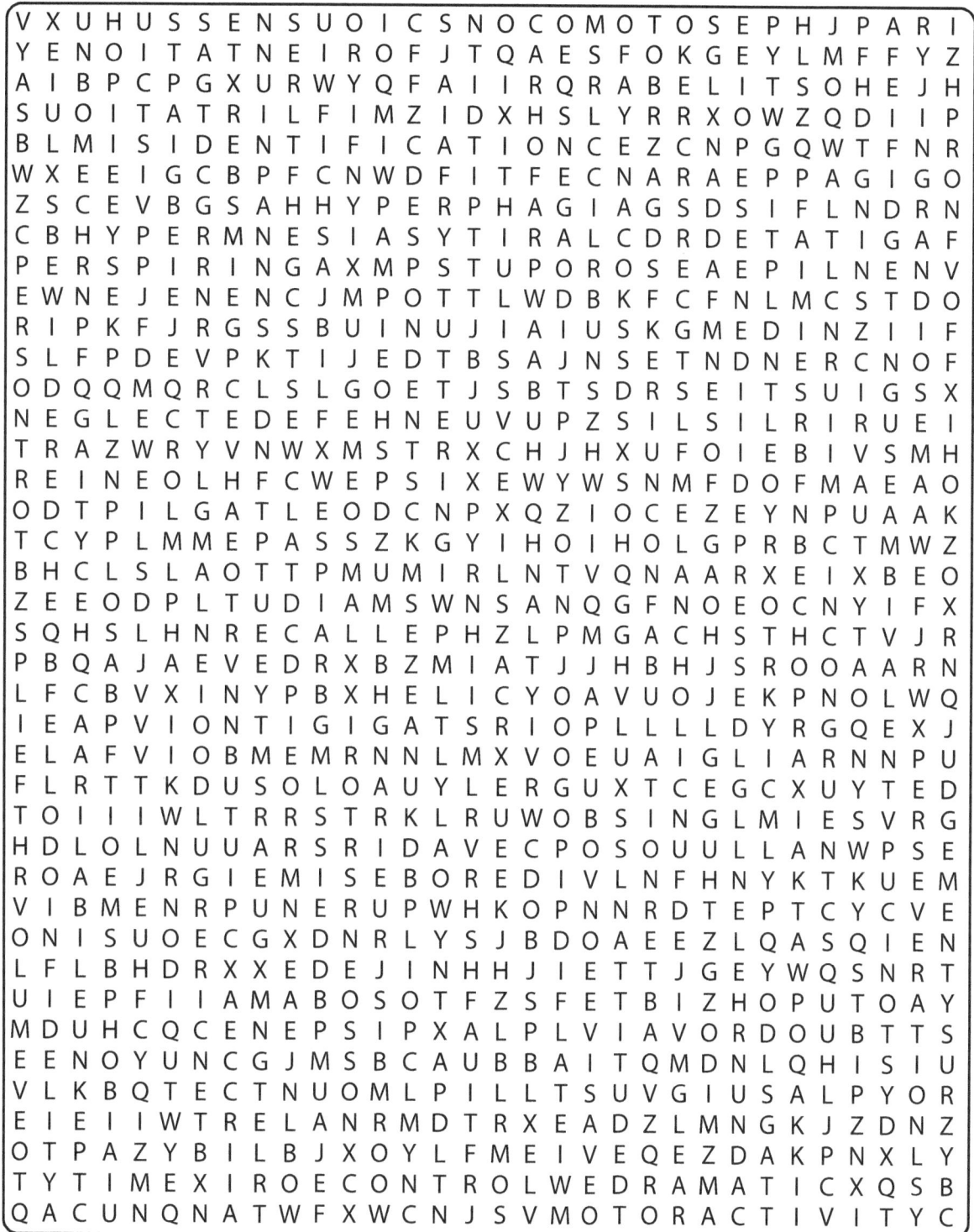

**Figure 8.2:** Mental Status Word Search—Recalling Words Related to Assessing Risk

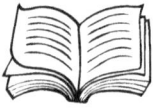

## STUDY QUESTIONS

**1.** What four areas must be assessed to determine a person's level of risk?

_____

_____

_____

_____

**2.** If a person has suicidal or homicidal ideation, what are five follow-up questions that need to be asked?

_____

_____

_____

_____

_____

_____

_____

**3.** How does a clinician determine if a person is experiencing delusional thought content?

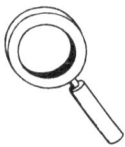

_____

_____

_____

_____

_____

## CASE STUDY

Sam is a 20-year-old male who has dealt with repeated bouts of depression since he was 16. He also has colitis, which has never been controlled well. His gastroenterologist is recommending that he have surgery. He had thought his depression was in remission, but over the last three months his depressive symptoms have been escalating. When feeling low, he self-medicates with marijuana and alcohol. Three weeks ago, Sam and his long-term girlfriend of two years broke up. She told him that she just couldn't watch him go through another depression bout; it was too hard on her. He suspected that she was seeing someone else because she had become secretive with her plans and more distant. It really wasn't a surprise that she wanted to break up.

Sam had never heard voices before. Shortly after the breakup, he started to hear a woman's voice telling him that he was worthless. Over the last three weeks, the voice has become louder and more insistent. The voice tells Sam that he is a loser, that any dreams he has of becoming an artist are a joke, and that everyone would be better off if he were dead. Over the last week, the woman's voice repeatedly tells him that he just doesn't "have what it takes" to kill himself. Sam thought about death before the breakup, but now he thinks about it every day. The intensity of the thoughts is increasing. The voice tells him to "go and shoot himself." He doesn't want to but states, "This [voice] is driving me crazy." Sam is afraid that the voice will make him do something he doesn't want to do. He asks for your help.

## Case Study Activity: What's the Risk?

Based on the case study above, use table 8.1 to identify what risk factors are present, what evidence you are basing this decision on, and what strategy can be used to reduce the effect of the identified risk factor.

**Table 8.1:** What's the Risk?

| Circle the risk factors that are present in the above case study. | Identify the phrases in the case study that support this decision. | Identify a strategy that can be used to reduce the effect of the risk factor. |
|---|---|---|
| *Psychiatric illness* | | |
| *Medical illness* | | |
| *Life stressors* | | |
| *Substance use* | | |
| *Personality disorder* | | |

*continued*

| | | |
|---|---|---|
| *Suicidal behaviour* | | |
| *Psychological vulnerability* | | |
| *Hopelessness* | | |
| *Family history* | | |

# REFERENCES

Soole, R., Kolves, K., & De Leo, D. (2015). Suicide in children: A systematic review. *Archives of Suicide Research*, *19*(3), 285–304. doi:10.1080/13811118.2014.996694

World Health Organization. (2014). *Preventing suicide: A global imperative*. Geneva, Switzerland: World Health Organization.

# CHAPTER 9

## Perception

**Photo 9.1:** Shadow Pipers

> A hallucination is a fact, not an error; what is erroneous is a judgment based upon it.
> —*Bertrand Russell*

## LEARNING OBJECTIVES

**At the completion of this chapter, the reader will be able to:**

- identify the major categories within the perception component of the psychiatric mental status examination
- describe assessment indicators for hallucinations, illusions, misidentification, and depersonalization

- document objective and subjective assessment findings
- define key terms that may be used in this section of the psychiatric mental status examination
- identify how culture and age affect the assessment of perception

# HOW IS PERCEPTION ASSESSED?

In this portion of the mental status examination, the client's sensory perceptions are assessed. A person may experience a hallucination with any one of the senses: auditory, visual, gustatory, tactile, olfactory, proprioception, kinesthetic, and somatic. The experience of hearing voices should not be confused with the inner voice that we all have in our minds when we are in good mental health. The content, mode of onset, source, vividness, reality of experience, and time of the hallucination should be assessed. In addition, the circumstances in which hallucinations occur, their persistence and frequency, and their effects on the individual, as well as the individual's use of coping mechanisms and their effectiveness should be explored and documented. The presence of command hallucinations is associated with increased risk, and should prompt further intensive risk assessment (as discussed in chapter 8).

Usually the client describes the perceptual disturbances; however, when they do not report abnormal perceptions, but in the clinician's judgment the client's general behaviour suggests that they are having hallucinations, a notation about this behaviour should be made.

**Table 9.1:** Categories of Perceptual Disturbance

| Categories of perceptual disturbance | Description |
| --- | --- |
| *Hallucination* | Hallucinations are sensory perceptions in the absence of an external stimulus. They may involve bodily sensations, such as deadness, pain, or other tactile feelings, or may involve the special senses—auditory, visual, olfactory, or gustatory. |
| | Hallucinations may be normal if they occur when the patient is falling asleep or waking from sleep; these hallucinations are referred to as hypnagogic and hypnopompic, respectively. |
| *Illusion* | Illusions are misinterpretations of actual external events and may involve the same sensory modalities as hallucinations. The distinction between hallucinations and illusions is important, as hallucinations are more often indicators of serious psychiatric disturbance than are illusions. |

| Misidentification | Misidentification occurs when individuals falsely believe they recognize a sound, person, taste, or object. |
|---|---|
| Depersonalization | Depersonalization is a sense of unreality, estrangement, or detachment from your body or environment. For example, a person who is hallucinating may feel an arm is shrunken or distorted in some way, but this arm still feels like it is part of the person's body. A person who is experiencing depersonalization may also experience the sense that the arm is shrunken or distorted, but they also experience that this body part is not really attached to their body or a feeling like they are living in a dream. |

## How Do You Ask a Person If They Are Hallucinating?

There are four main categories of perceptual disturbances: hallucinations, illusions, misidentification, and depersonalization. Hallucinations are about an individual experiencing something that others do not. To investigate hallucinations, the clinician needs to make a determination regarding the presence of an external stimulus. It is useful to begin with a general question, such as, "Do you ever experience things that others do not?" If the answer is yes, or the client responds with "What do you mean?" you may choose to elaborate by asking, "Have you ever seen or heard things that others do not?" As auditory and visual hallucinations are most common, most clinicians start with these examples. The following questions are examples that can be used to help you gather more information about hallucinations. You can alter the questions (for example, changing "What do they say?" to "What do you see?"), so that they are appropriate for the type of hallucination you are exploring.

- Do your thoughts ever feel so intense that they sound like a voice?
- How many different voices do you hear?
- Tell me what the voices sound like to you. Can you hear them clearly? Are they mumbling?
- What do they say?
- Do they say mean things about you or others?
- Are they male or female?
- Do they seem to come from inside your head or do they come from outside your head?
- How loud are they?
- When you first heard the voices what did you think they were?
- What feelings do you have when you hear the voices?
- Have you ever noticed smells that other people do not?
- Have you ever had a sensation on or under your skin that didn't make sense to you?
- Have you been seeing visions?

## How Do You Ask If a Person Experiences Illusions?

An illusion differs from a hallucination because an illusion results from external stimulus. An illusion is a perception of something in a way that causes a misinterpretation of what is perceived. Accompanying an illusion is a firmness of belief that what is perceived is the true representation of the object. For example, an illusion is experienced when you feel a huge spider on your arm and look down to realize it is tree branch that has brushed your arm. Common illusions include misperceiving a shadow, movement of a curtain, plants in the corner, or a coat stand as a person. The following are sample questions you can use to start assessing the presence of illusions.

- Have you ever looked at an image or object and then seen it change?
- Have you ever thought you heard someone call your name, but then realized you must have been mistaken?
- Have you ever had an experience in which you thought you saw something, but when you looked, nothing was there?
- Have you ever felt something on your skin, then realized that it was an itch?
- Have you ever been so hungry that it felt like you could taste food in your mouth?

## How Do You Ask If a Person Experiences Misidentification?

When assessing for misidentification, the clinician looks for symptoms related to disorders of recognition (agnosias). These symptoms occur when there are impairments with perceptual integration. When assessing for misidentification, the following questions are a useful place to start. It is important to remember that there are many types of misidentification and that they can involve all of the senses.

- Do you have difficulty recognizing faces?
- What is this called? (Clinician points to an object in the room, such as a clock or chair, when asking this question.)

## How Do You Ask If a Person Experiences Depersonalization?

Depersonalization is a sense that you are detached from your body. These symptoms can be difficult to describe. What clients report is often vague, but they are sure that something is wrong. As a clinician, you are assessing for a sense of separation. The following sample questions that can be used to assess the client for depersonalization.

- Have you ever felt disconnected from your body?
- Have you walked into a room in your home and it was unfamiliar to you?

- Have you ever felt like you were living in a movie?
- Have you ever felt like you were numb (emotionally or physically) and not able to feel anything?
- Have you looked in the mirror and felt detached?
- Does it feel like your memories belong to someone else?

# HOW DO YOU DOCUMENT PERCEPTION?

Documenting perception is about capturing the individual's experiences. Most of this documentation describes what the individual reports. Occasionally, it also describes behaviours that the clinician believes are in response to a perceptual disturbance. Box 9.1 provides examples of documentation.

## BOX 9.1: DOCUMENTING INFORMATION ABOUT THOUGHT CONTENT

### Nora

The client denies any perceptual disturbances.

### Rodney

He did indicate that there are times that he sees bugs in the room. This is not frequent; however, he does worry about it. Rodney is scanning the room. He focuses on one of the floor tiles. His eyes move back and forth as if following something. Rodney draws his legs under the chair and lifts his feet. When asked if he is seeing any bugs now, he yells, "No!"

### Kia

Almost every day Kia reports feeling like there are bugs crawling under her skin. She has tried to remove them herself but has never found a real bug. These sensations occur most frequently when Kia doesn't have enough money to buy liquor.

### Mrs. Gee

Over the past month, Mrs. Gee has become increasingly upset and worried about the man who is trying to sneak through her window. Mrs. Gee has called the police on three separate occasions to report a break-in. The police have always had to be let into the house as the door was locked. They have never found any evidence of a break-in. Mrs. Gee's daughter has stayed overnight at her mother's home on several occasions. One night, she was awoken by her mother screaming, "Get out, get out!" Mrs. Gee's daughter reports that her mother was yelling at the curtains that were moving slightly over the air vent. Mrs. Gee's daughter reports that all the

*continued*

curtains have been removed from her mom's bedroom. Since that time her mother has not reported any other break-ins or suspicious activity around her home.

## SPECIAL CONSIDERATIONS

If there are perceptual disturbances present, when assessing perception, it is important to explore if there are times that they occur with less intensity or frequency. It is also important to investigate how bothersome these experiences are to the client. Children may have imaginary friends that they see and talk with. Developmental age is an important consideration when determining if a finding is expected, a common variation, or unexpected and in need of further investigation. It is commonly reported that people who have recently lost a loved one will continue to hear their voice after they have died. In some cultures, hearing voices or seeing visions is accepted and valued as a religious or spiritual experience. When experiencing voices or visions within this context, they are often benign or friendly. Those who experience perceptual alterations as part of a psychotic disorder will often experience deprecating sensations.

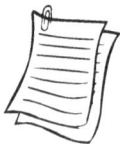

## CHAPTER GLOSSARY TERMS

**auditory hallucination:** A sound that does not have a concrete, external stimulus. For some people who hear voices, the voices will be clear, whereas for others they may sound like a constant mumbling in the background. Some people hear only one voice, while others may hear a number of different voices at the same time.

**command hallucination:** A unique kind of auditory hallucination in which a voice that is giving instructions to a person does not have a concrete, external stimulus.

**gustatory hallucination:** A taste that does not have a concrete external stimulus.

**hallucinations:** Sensory perceptions that do not have a concrete external stimulus.

**illusions:** Misinterpretations of actual sensory stimuli. Illusions should be carefully distinguished from hallucinations. Illusions may occur in any sensory modality.

**kinesthetic hallucination:** A sensation that a body part is moving without a concrete, external stimulus.

**olfactory hallucination:** A smell that does not have a concrete external stimulus.

**proprioceptive hallucination:** A sensation of body posture without a concrete external stimulus. For example, a sensation that you are floating, when you are actually lying in your bed.

**somatic hallucination:** A physical experience that something is happening within the body without a concrete, external stimulus.

**tactile hallucination:** A feeling that does not have a concrete, external stimulus.

**visual hallucination:** Seeing something that does not have a concrete, external stimulus.

# ACTIVITY: WHAT IS EXPECTED VERSUS UNEXPECTED?

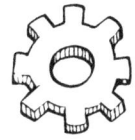

Complete table 9.2 and identify expected findings, common variations, and unexpected findings for each of the senses.

**Table 9.2:** Perceptual Variation Table

| Assessment area | Expected findings | Common variations | Unexpected findings/ further assessment required |
|---|---|---|---|
| **Hearing** | | | Auditory hallucination |
| | | | Auditory illusion |
| | | | Auditory misidentification |
| **Vision** | | | Visual hallucination |
| | | | Visual illusion |
| | | | Visual misidentification |

*continued*

| | | | |
|---|---|---|---|
| **Taste** | | | Gustatory hallucination |
| | | | Gustatory illusion |
| | | | Gustatory misidentification |
| **Touch** | | | Tactile hallucination |
| | | | Tactile illusion |
| | | | Tactile misidentification |
| **Smell** | | | Olfactory hallucination |
| | | | Olfactory illusion |
| | | | Olfactory misidentification |

| *Experience of surroundings* | | | Depersonalization |
|---|---|---|---|
| | | | |

## STUDY QUESTIONS

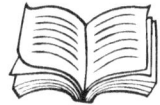

**1.** What are the four categories of perceptual disturbances?

_____
_____
_____
_____

**2.** What is a tactile hallucination? How is this different than a tactile misidentification? How is this different than a tactile illusion?

_____
_____
_____
_____
_____
_____
_____
_____

## CASE STUDY

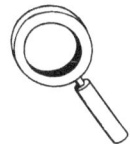

Pilan is an Indigenous 23-year-old male. He has lived with his grandparents since he was two years old. His grandfather is a recognized leader in the community who knows the "old ways." Pilan tells you that his grandfather is a powerful medicine man who has been teaching Pilan about Indigenous medicine. People come to see his grandfather for help with medical problems and other problems in their lives. Four months ago, Pilan went on his first vision quest. In preparing for the quest, he prayed, ate sacred foods, and ingested sacred herbs. On the quest, he met the Little People who shared their secrets with him. They told him that he would be even more powerful than his grandfather. He was going to be a great man. Since returning from his quest, Pilan continues to feel the spiritual healing powers within himself; he can hear animals talk to him and can see messages written in the wind.

Pilan was recently arrested after chasing a woman in a train station. He reports that he was only trying to tell her that she needed to be careful because the spirits revealed to him that she was in danger.

## Case Study Questions

1. Identify which of Pilan's experiences are unexpected and need further assessment.

_____

_____

_____

_____

2. What are three strategies that can be used to determine if there was an external stimulus for Pilan's experiences?

_____

_____

_____

_____

3. What three strategies can be used by health care providers to balance the benefits of belief and its ability to do harm?

_____

_____

_____

_____

_____

_____

_____

# CHAPTER 10

## Cognitive State

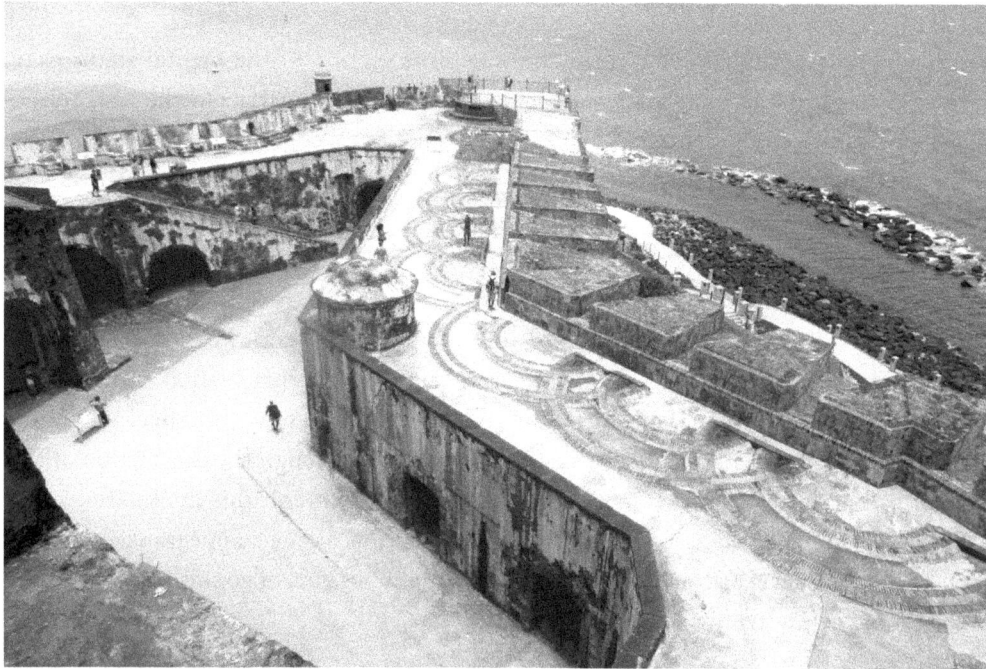

**Photo 10.1:** Finding Your Way

The true art of memory is the art of attention.
—*Samuel Johnson*

## LEARNING OBJECTIVES

**At the completion of this chapter, the reader will be able to:**

- identify the major categories within the cognitive state/sensorium component of the psychiatric mental status examination
- describe assessment indicators for abstract thinking, intellectual ability, judgment, general information, memory, concentration and attention, orientation, and consciousness

- document objective and subjective assessment findings
- define key terms that may be used in this section of the psychiatric mental status examination
- identify how culture and age may affect the assessment of mood and affect

# HOW IS COGNITIVE STATE/SENSORIUM ASSESSED?

Cognition reflects higher cortical functioning. This section of the mental status exam involves an assessment of awareness, alertness, and ability to carry out the tests related to general knowledge, orientation, memory, attention, and concentration, as well as the ability to think abstractly and demonstrate social judgment. This section of the mental status exam is sometimes referred to as *sensorium*. Some clinicians will complete only this portion of the mental status exam. When this is done, it is referred to as a mini–mental state exam (MMSE).

In contrast to the other sections of the mental status exam, cognition is tested in a structured manner. There are eight categories within this section of the exam: consciousness, orientation, concentration and attention, memory, intellectual ability, general information, judgment, and abstract thinking. Although the description of this section of the mental status comes more than halfway through this book, after interviewing your client and assessing a general description of their appearance, you will then assess their level of consciousness. The other components of cognition are assessed throughout the interview.

## Consciousness

Consciousness describes the individual's level of awareness of self and the environment. Characteristics that are associated with higher levels of consciousness are an ability to follow instructions, the ability to communicate, and purposeful movement. The description of level of consciousness for the purposes of a mental status exam is very general. Specific level of consciousness measures or coma scale levels are generally not reported; instead, the clinician would document that the individual was alert, drowsy, delirious, stuperose, comatose, or had fluctuating levels of consciousness. When assessing consciousness, the clinician needs to consider factors that may affect a person's responses, such as drug use, alcohol intoxication, shock, or other medical conditions, including low blood sugar, low blood oxygen, and altered serum electrolytes. If an individual has a very low level of consciousness, it is not possible to complete the rest of the mental status examination.

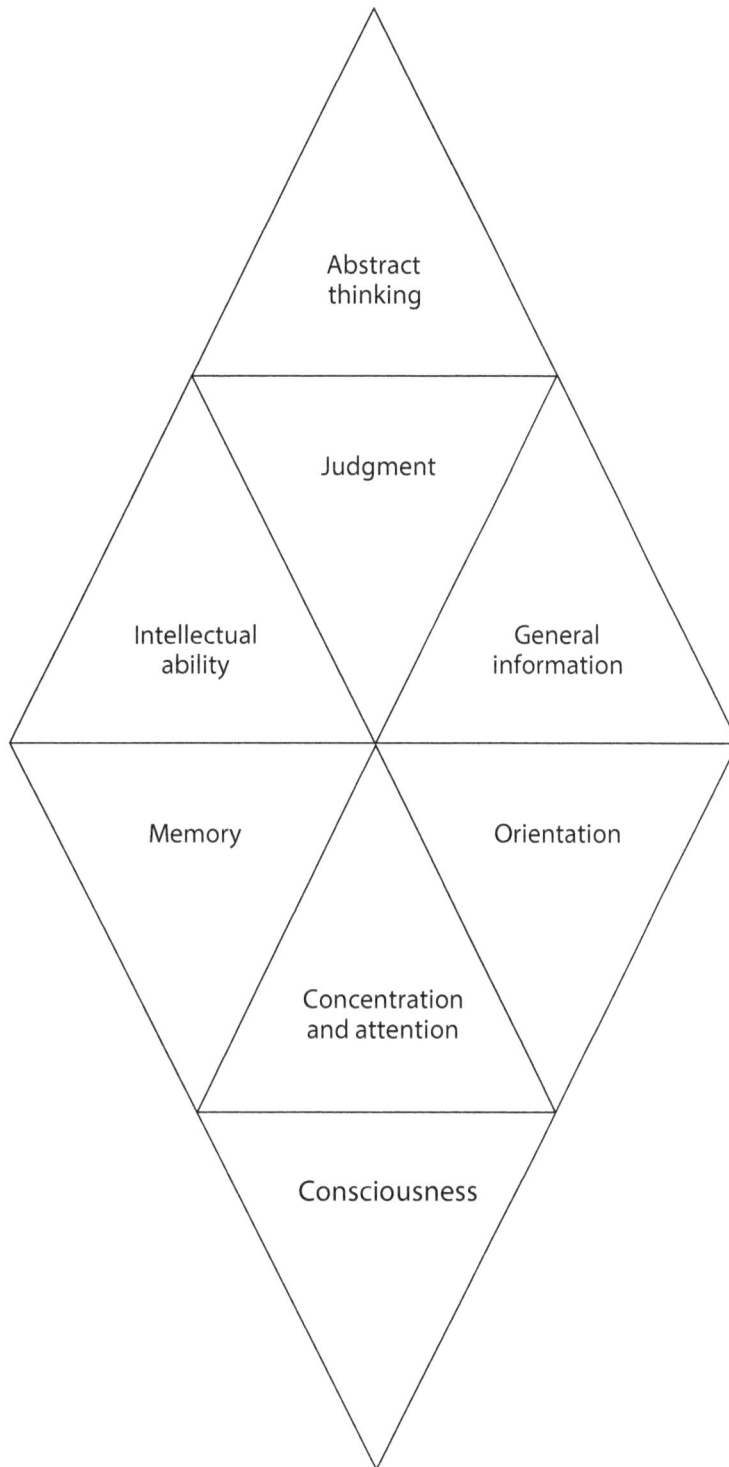

**Figure 10.1:** Components of Cognitive State Assessment

## Orientation

Orientation relates to an individual's ability to determine direction or position of the self and their environment. Essentially, orientation means to be acquainted with a situation and the surrounding environment. People who are oriented can recognize themselves and others. They can also determine where they are and when (for example, morning or afternoon, how old they are, what year it is). Orientation is evaluated based on a person's ability to determine time, place, and person. Several conversational questions can be used to assess orientation. For example, place can be assessed by asking: Did you have any trouble finding the office today? How did you get here today? or Where did you park? Other questions that can be used to assess time, place, and person are listed below.

- Time: Does the person have an awareness of movement?
  - What is today's date?
  - What day of the week is it?
  - What time is it?
  - What month is it?
  - What season is it?
  - Are there times when you seem to lose track of time?
- Place: Does the person know where they are?
  - What type of building are we in now?
  - What is the purpose of this building?
  - What goes on in this building?
  - What floor are we on?
- Person: Does the person know who they are, and do they recognize their relationship with the clinician?
  - What is your full name?
  - What is my name? What is my job?
  - Who is this person in the mirror? (Clinician holds up a small mirror in front of the client.)

For people with neurocognitive disorders, disorientation to time usually occurs before disorientation to place. Orientation to person is maintained the longest.

## Concentration and Attention

Concentration is the ability to sustain attention. Attention is the ability to direct mental energy. Changes in concentration and attention affect a person's ability to store and access memories, and their ability to follow instructions. Assessing these areas involves determining how easily the person can manipulate information. For example, attention can be assessed by asking the person to spell a word backwards; however, it is important to ensure that the person knows how to spell the word correctly before doing so. As a clinician, you can also use a digit span test to assess concentration. Start by listing four random numbers for the client, then ask the client to repeat these numbers. If they are correct, ask them to repeat these numbers backwards. Most adults can repeat 5 to 7 digits in this manner without error.

Concentration can also be assessed throughout the interview. Clinicians will ask themselves if the client follows the conversation and is able to hold a focused discussion. If further assessment is needed, a more structured way to assess concentration is to use subtraction or addition. A common serial subtraction is serial sevens. The client is asked to start from 100 and subtract 7 (100 − 7, 93 − 7 …) until they get to zero. Another commonly used serial subtraction is serial threes. The client is asked to start at 20 and subtract 3 (20 − 3, 17 − 3 …) until they get to zero. Mathematical ability is also assessed when serial numeric questions are used; therefore, the level of difficulty should correspond to the person's education level. The person should be able to answer the questions.

## Memory

For the purposes of the mental status exam, memory is divided into immediate retention or registration, recent memory or short-term recall, and long-term memory or long-term recall. Each of these functions should be tested separately in any client with whom there is a suspicion of impairment. If you have used a digit span to assess attention, this has also assessed registration. Registration or immediate memory is most affected when there are changes in concentration and attention. Recent memory can be generally assessed by asking the person what activities they did earlier in the day, such as what they had for breakfast (if these facts can be verified). It is sometimes useful at the end of the interview to ask the client if they remember your name or some other event that happened earlier in the interview, as these will be part of their recent memory period. Long-term memory can be assessed by asking the client about important events that occurred when they were younger or before their current illness or disease.

## Intellectual Ability

This is not tested directly, but is determined by the individual's use of vocabulary, logic, problem-solving abilities, symbolism, and ability to assimilate information. When assessing a client's approximate intelligence, contributing factors include general knowledge, education level, and occupational records. If you notice a wide disparity between the client's previous cognitive functioning and abilities from assessment of orientation, concentration and attention, and present general information, this should be noted.

## General Information

General information, sometimes referred to as general information fund, is related to the individual's level of common knowledge. Questions in this component of cognition need to be developed after considering the person's educational level, experiences, and interests. Sample questions include being able to name the current prime minister and governing political party, the premier of the province, the capital city, and so on. When assessing children, questions may be related to the name of their favourite character and what story they are from or a specific sports team.

## Judgment

Judgment is a process of forming an opinion or conclusion based on information about a situation that can lead to a decision or action. It is an assessment of real-life problem-solving skills with the recognition of associated consequences. Social judgment may be largely assessed during the person's history. Judgment may be tested by asking the individual what they would do in an imaginary situation; for example, what would you do if you were sitting in a crowded theatre and smelled smoke? Asking questions more pertinent to the person's illness is often more helpful. The clinician could ask the following: How do you think your hallucinations should be handled? What are you planning on doing after you are discharged from the hospital? A person's follow-through with agreed upon treatment plans is also a good indication of judgment.

## Abstract Thinking

The capacity for abstract thinking is the ability to generalize and describe similarities; these are lateral thinking skills, sometimes referred to as fluid intelligence. This area of thinking is assessed by asking an individual how two objects are alike, for example, "How are a mosquito and a flower alike?" A good response is, "They are both alive"; a poor response is "Nothing." This area can also be tested by asking the client to interpret a proverb. For example, "People in glass houses shouldn't throw stones." A good response is, "Don't criticize others for faults that you have in yourself"; a poor response is, "It is bad to break glass." Box 10.1 provides further examples of responses that suggest normal ability to think in the abstract, concreteness of thought, or bizarre thinking.

## BOX 10.1: ABSTRACT THINKING INTERPRETATION

**Proverb Interpretation**
"A stitch in time saves nine."

- Abstract interpretation: "A little prevention can save a lot of work."

- Concrete interpretation: "When your shirt has a tear in it, you should put a stitch in it or you may end up having to put many stitches in it."
- Bizarre interpretation: "I laughed and laughed and laughed until I was in stitches."

### Similarity Interpretation

"How are an apple and an orange similar?"

- Abstract interpretation: "They are both fruit."
- Concrete interpretation: "They are both round."
- Bizarre interpretation: "I eat and eat them to turn into a pumpkin."

---

When there are unexpected variations, further assessment is required. The most commonly used screening tools are the mini–mental state exam (Folstein, Folstein, & McHugh, 1975) and the Montreal cognitive assessment (Nasreddine et al., 2005), which assess orientation, memory, calculations, reading and writing capacity, visuospatial ability, and language.

There are many different illnesses that affect an individual's cognition; therefore, it is important that the findings of this portion of the mental status exam are documented. Box 10.2 provides examples of documentation for cognition. When screening tools are used, the tools used and the score the client obtained should be documented. Areas of strength and weakness should also be highlighted.

## BOX 10.2: DOCUMENTING COGNITION FINDINGS

### George

George was alert and oriented to time, place, and person. He could answer questions and recall significant past events without difficulty.

### Max

Max is alert and oriented to time, place, and person. Questions had to be repeated several times. He reports having difficulty concentrating and paying attention. Max completed graduate school in mathematics, but feels like he is unable to recall even the most basic information. Despite the reports of poor memory, Max has a good general information fund and could recount important events from his childhood and adult life. With effort, he could recall what he had for breakfast. Immediate recall, though, is poor. He was unable to repeat back four digits in reverse order. Although he describes himself as a concrete thinker, he had no difficulties interpreting proverbs. Max identifies that he is not himself and believes he has depression.

*continued*

**Mrs. Adamowski**

Mrs. Adamowski had fluctuating levels of consciousness during the interview. At times, she could respond to questions, but then would seem to fall asleep mid-response. She was unable to recall where she was, but stated that she thought she was in the hospital but did not know why she was there. She was unable to complete serial threes and had a two-digit span of recall. A Folstein's MMSE was completed. She scored 15 out of 30. In addition to problems with orientation, she had difficulty with calculations, following a three-stage command, visuospatial ability, and language; however, she was consistently oriented to person.

## SPECIAL CONSIDERATIONS

When assessing cognition, its components are interrelated. When there are variations, it is essential that for the clinician to view the person in a holistic manner and consider developmental, cultural, educational, and social factors that affect the results of the assessment. Abstraction depends on the level of intelligence, insight and judgment, and education. As a result, abstraction is a relative concept. Abstraction abilities vary according to age. For example, "the day after tomorrow" is a highly abstract concept for a two-year-old. For an adolescent, "the day after tomorrow" is relatively concrete.

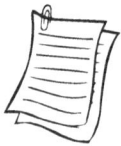

## CHAPTER GLOSSARY TERMS

**abstract thinking:** The ability to generalize thinking and form ideas that are part of an instance or material objects, but are not concrete.

**amnesia:** Disturbance in memory manifested by partial or total inability to recall past experiences.

**attention:** The aspect of consciousness that relates to the amount of effort exerted in focusing on certain aspects of an experience. It is sometimes used interchangeably with *concentration*.

**clouding of consciousness:** Disturbance of consciousness characterized by unclear sensory perceptions due to diminished alertness and apparent inability to concentrate.

**confabulation:** Retrospective falsification of memory

**confusion:** Diminished alertness and awareness and impaired sensorium; difficulty grasping a situation, accompanied by disorientation with regard to time, place, and person.

**delirium:** Disturbance in the state of consciousness stemming from an organic reaction characterized by restlessness, confusion, disorientation, bewilderment, agitation, and affective lability.

**dementia:** An older term used to indicate organic loss of mental functioning. The current diagnostic term is *major neurocognitive disorder.*

**hypermnesia:** Exaggerated degree of retention and recall. It is observed sometimes in schizophrenia, manic drug intoxications, and hypnosis.

**judgment:** The mental act of comparing or evaluating choices within the framework of a given set of values to select a course of action. Judgment is said to be intact if the course of action is consistent with reality.

**orientation:** The ability to identify oneself with respect to one's position in time, place, and person.

**paramnesia:** Disturbance of memory in which reality and fantasy are confused.

**perplexity:** A pervasive feeling of bewilderment and uncertainty.

**perseveration:** Pathological repetition of the same response to different questions.

## ACTIVITY: WHAT IS EXPECTED VERSUS UNEXPECTED?

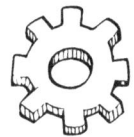

Complete table 10.1 and compare expected findings to common variations and unexpected findings.

**Table 10.1:** Cognitive State/Sensorium Variation Table

| Assessment area | Expected findings | Common variations | Unexpected findings/ further assessment required |
|---|---|---|---|
| *Consciousness* | | | |
| *Orientation* | | | |

*continued*

| | | | |
|---|---|---|---|
| **Concentration and attention** | | | |
| **Memory** | | | |
| **Intellectual ability** | | | |
| **General information** | | | |
| **Judgment** | | | |
| **Abstract thinking** | | | |

## STUDY QUESTIONS

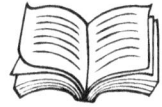

**1.** What are the eight components of cognition?

_____
_____
_____
_____
_____
_____

**2.** How does a mini–mental state exam vary from a mental status examination?

_____
_____
_____
_____

**3.** What is the best way to assess judgment? Why?

_____
_____
_____
_____

## CASE STUDY

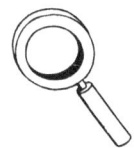

Mrs. Adamowski was admitted to hospital for a bowel resection. Upon admission, she discussed her advanced directives with the unit social worker. During this conversation, she also identified how anxious she was about the surgery, and said that if anything happened, her husband would not be able to make the decisions that were needed. Mrs. Adamowski was very specific about her desire for no heroic measures. When completing the admission assessment, the social worker completed a Folstein's MMSE. Mrs. Adamowski scored 30 out of 30.

After the surgery, Mrs. Adamowski was in a significant amount of pain. She was given pain medication every four hours. Her husband stayed at her bedside. He was becoming increasingly concerned because she was beginning to make no sense. She was referring to him as her father, didn't know where she was, and flipped from English to Ukrainian. He was about to get the nurse when she fell asleep. After she awoke, she seemed okay when the doctor visited, but within half an hour she was once again not making any sense. She had an exaggerated startle response when she heard the call bells from the other clients' rooms and then started to yell, "Those kids they know better than to play in the car."

You come to see Mrs. Adamowski two days after her surgery. Her arms are restrained as she has been pulling out her intravenous infusion lines. When you introduce yourself, she says hello and asks if you can help, as she is thirsty and would like a drink. She tries to smooth her hair and says apologetically, "I must look a mess." She is unable to recall where she is, but says she thinks she is in a hospital but does not know why. You complete a Folstein's MMSE. She scores 15 out of 30. In addition to problems with orientation, she has difficulty with calculations, following a three-stage command, visuospatial ability, and language; however, she is consistently oriented to person.

## Case Study Question

Using the evidence provided in the case study, complete table 10.2.

**Table 10.2:** What Do You See?

|  | Finding | Evidence provided in the case study |
|---|---|---|
| *Onset* | Sudden acute onset | Admission: Folstein's mini–mental state exam (MMSE) 30/30. Two days later: MMSE 15/30. |
| *Consciousness* | Fluctuates |  |
| *Awareness* | Unaware of condition<br><br>May experience hallucinations or delusions |  |

| | | |
|---|---|---|
| **Motor behaviour** | Varies between hypo- and hyper arousal | |
| **Mood** | Anxious<br><br>Restless<br><br>Mixed hallucinations and illusions | |
| **Affect** | Fluctuating and nonsensical inter-actions with others | |
| **Physical** | Acute medical illness<br><br>Drug reaction | |
| **Memory** | Fluctuating performance<br><br>Forgets most of experience | |
| **Sleep** | Behaviour disorders worsen at night | |

*continued*

| | | |
|---|---|---|
| *Self-care* | Often unable to perform activities of daily living (ADLs) | |

# REFERENCES

Folstein, M. F., Folstein, S. E., & McHugh, P. R. (1975). Mini–mental state: A practical method for grading the cognitive state of patients for the clinician. *Journal of Psychiatric Research, 12*(3), 189–198.

Nasreddin, Z. S., Phillips, N. A., Bedirian, V., Charbonneau, S., Whitehead, V., Collin, I., Cummings, J. L., & Chertkow, H. (2005). The Montreal cognitive assessment, MoCA: A brief screening tool for mild cognitive impairment. *Journal of the American Geriatrics Society, 53*(4), 695–699. doi:10.1111/j.1532-5415.2005.53221.x

# CHAPTER 11

## Insight

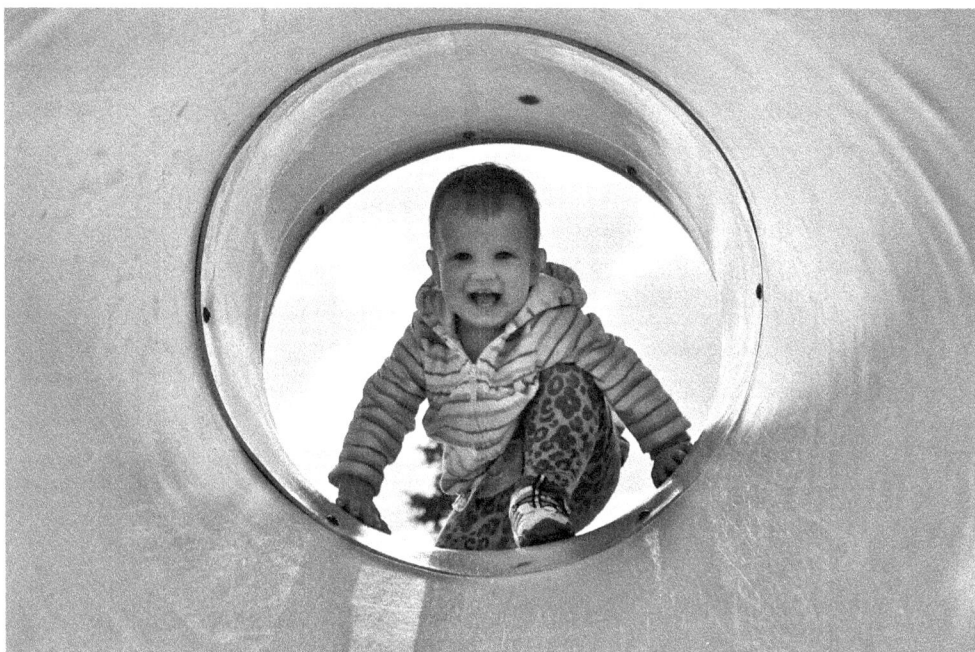

**Photo 11.1:** Understand Where You Are

> A point of view can be a dangerous luxury when substituted for insight and understanding.
> —*Marshall McLuhan*

## LEARNING OBJECTIVES

**At the completion of this chapter, the reader will be able to:**

- discuss the continuum of insight
- describe assessment indicators for insight
- document objective and subjective assessment findings
- define key terms that may be used in this section of the psychiatric mental status examination
- identify how culture and age may affect the assessment of insight

# HOW IS INSIGHT ASSESSED?

Insight involves the capacity to examine many aspects, viewpoints, and consequences of an issue before forming an opinion or making a decision. Intact cognitive functioning alone is not adequate to have good insight; a person must also be able to think conceptually and abstractly. Insight may be affected by a person's intellectual ability, cognitive function, defence mechanisms, personality style, presence or absence of a thought disorder, and cultural context. In the context of the mental status examination, assessment of insight focuses on three factors: first, the person's self-awareness that there is a problem or illness; second, the non-delusional understanding of its cause or meaning; and third, understanding of the potential effects of treatment. Understanding the potential effects of treatment requires the person to consider the interplay between personal weaknesses and sensitivities, personal strengths, and the severity of the illness.

To assess insight, the clinician will ask, "What do you think is the problem?" and "Do you think there is anything that will help you feel better?" Many other questions can also be used to assess insight (see box 11.1). Responses will fall along a continuum that ranges from denial to awareness of illness and attributing illness to correct causes.

## BOX 11.1: QUESTIONS TO EXPLORE INSIGHT

- How do you feel?
- Do you feel ill?
- Do you ever experience things that aren't really there or that seem strange?
- What is the cause of these experiences? Is it internal or external?
- Do you ever see things that other people cannot?
- Do you hear voices or sounds when there is nothing around to explain them?
- Do you think that you need help to reduce or eliminate these experiences?
- Do you need treatment? Why? How would it help?
- What type of treatment do you believe would be effective?
- How does this illness affect your life, your relationships, and/or your work?
- How bothered are you by your symptoms? How important is it to you that they are decreased or eliminated?

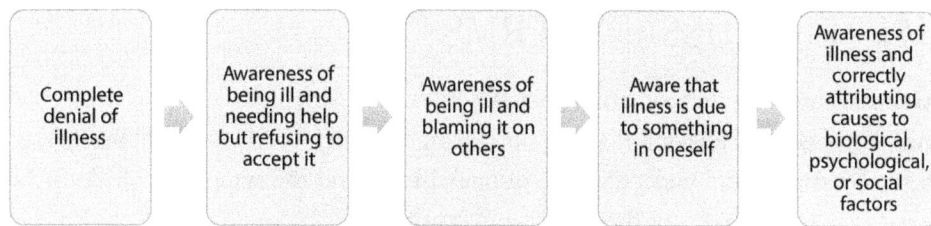

**Figure 11.1:** Insight Continuum

The evaluation of insight is important, as it provides the health care team with information that reflects how important treatment is to the client. If eliminating the symptoms is not important to the client, it is unlikely that they will actively engage in the prescribed treatment; however, if mutual goals can be established, there is a stronger therapeutic alliance and it is likely that the client will more closely follow the prescribed treatment. It is important to document the findings of your insight assessment, as this will facilitate the development of realistic treatment goals and outcomes. Box 11.2 provides examples of how to document insight findings.

## BOX 11.2: DOCUMENTING INSIGHT FINDINGS

### Aiden

Aiden identifies that he is depressed. He describes the depression as being caused by chemical changes in his brain and says that his medication helps to correct those changes.

### Meesha

Meesha describes herself as feeling different after she was raped. Since then, she has had difficulty concentrating, sleeping, and feeling anything. She describes cutting herself as a way to at least feel something. She believes that she needs help to deal with her feelings about the rape, but is not sure if anything will help.

# SPECIAL CONSIDERATIONS

Insight is a combination of self-awareness and understanding. As a result, clinicians must be aware of developmental milestones and must base their decisions about "normalcy" on expected hallmarks. For example, children may not have developed the ability to think conceptually and abstractly and, as a result, may attribute the cause of their problems to others or something magical.

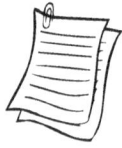

# CHAPTER GLOSSARY TERMS

**awareness:** Knowing that something exists.

**denial:** Erroneously believing that one's problem, difficulty, or illness is not present.

**insight:** Awareness and understanding of one's illness and the symptoms of illness, with or without an awareness of their cause and result.

# ACTIVITY: INSIGHT MATCHING EXERCISE

Insight is often linked to other findings of the mental status exam. The following activity provides a reminder of other sections that should also be considered when evaluating insight. Test your knowledge by completing the matching exercise below. Identify the correct definition for each of these words:

_____    affect

_____    general observations

_____    insight

_____    judgment

_____    memory

_____    mood

_____    orientation

_____    perceptions

_____    sensorium

_____    speech characteristics

_____    thinking

## Definitions

1. A client's wakefulness or consciousness. Levels of awareness include unconsciousness or coma, drowsiness or somnolence, normal alertness, and hyperalertness.

2. Observable characteristics of a person.

3. How the client is communicating, rather than what the client is telling you. Areas of evaluation include rate, volume, modulation, and flow.

4. A person's display of emotion or feelings.

5. The subjective way a client explains feelings.

6. The way the person functions intellectually; the process or way of thinking or analysis of the world; the way of connecting or associating thoughts; the overall organization of thoughts.

**7.** The way that a person experiences their environment and how they perceive their frame of reference within that environment. The information is perceived through the senses (vision, hearing, touch, smell, and taste) and monitored by the mind and its defences.

**8.** The mind's ability to recall events.

**9.** A person's ability to form valid conclusions and behave in a socially appropriate manner.

**10.** Level of awareness—the person's ability to identify who and where they are, the date, and the approximate time.

**11.** Awareness of one's own responsibilities and concerns, especially regarding their illness; a person's ability to analyze a problem objectively.

# STUDY QUESTIONS

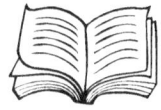

**1.** What are the three contributing factors that must be explored to assess insight?

_____

_____

_____

_____

**2.** Identify two questions that can be asked to explore each of the contributing factors of insight.

_____

_____

_____

_____

_____

**3.** Why is it important to document the assessment findings for insight?

_____

_____

_____

_____

_____

_____

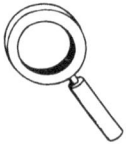

# CASE STUDY

Sam is a 20-year-old male who has dealt with repeated bouts of depression since he was 16. He also has colitis, which has never been controlled well. His gastroenterologist is recommending that he have surgery. He had thought his depression was in remission, but over the last three months his depressive symptoms have been escalating. When feeling low, he self-medicates with marijuana and alcohol. Three weeks ago, Sam and his long-term girlfriend of two years broke up. She told him that she just couldn't watch him go through another depression bout; it was too hard on her. He suspected that she was seeing someone else because she had become secretive with her plans and more distant. It really wasn't a surprise that she wanted to break up.

Sam had never heard voices before. Shortly after the breakup he started to hear a woman's voice telling him that he was worthless. Over the last three weeks, the voice has become louder and more insistent. The voice tells Sam that he is a loser, that any dreams he has of becoming an artist are a joke, and that everyone would be better off if he were dead. Over the last week, the woman's voice repeatedly tells him that he just doesn't "have what it takes" to kill himself. Sam thought about death before the breakup, but now he thinks about it every day. The intensity of the thoughts is increasing. The voice tells him to "go and shoot himself." He doesn't want to but states, "This [voice] is driving me crazy." Sam is afraid that the voice will make him do something he doesn't want to do. He asks for your help.

## Case Study Activity

Based on the case study above, complete table 11.1 and compare expected findings, common variations, and unexpected findings. Find examples of each in the case study.

**Table 11.1:** Variations in Insight: What Is Happening for Sam?

| Assessment area | Expected findings | Common variations | Unexpected findings/ further assessment required |
|---|---|---|---|
| *Awareness of Illness* | | | |

| | | | |
|---|---|---|---|
| *Cause of illness* | | | |
| *Understanding of the effects of treatment* | | | |

# CHAPTER 12

## Volition

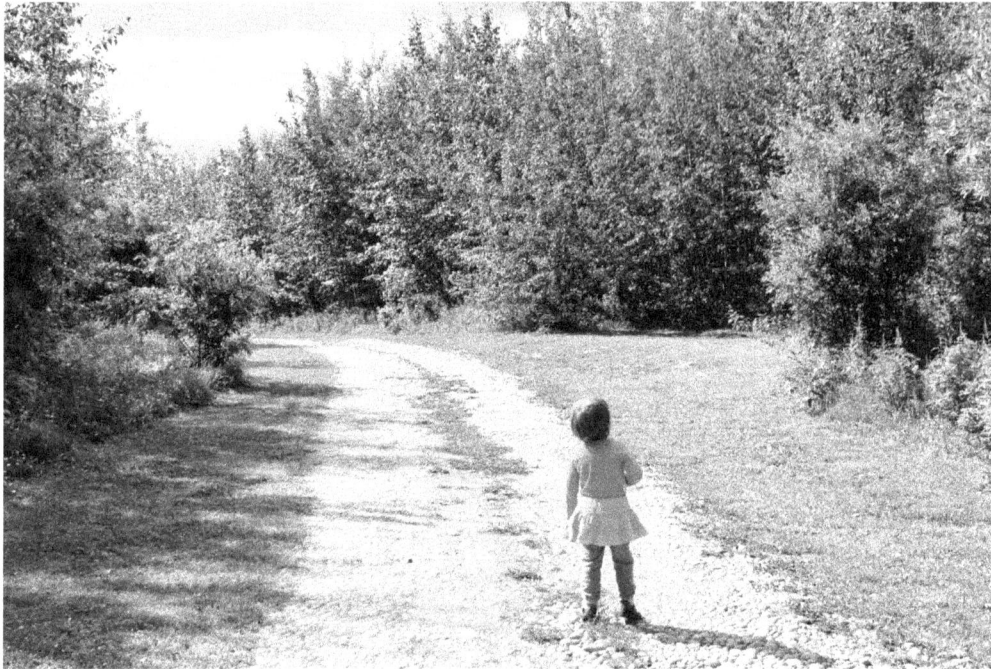

**Photo 12.1:** It's Still So Far Away

> A person with half volition goes backwards and forwards, but makes no progress on even the smoothest of roads.
> —*Thomas Carlyle*

## LEARNING OBJECTIVES

**At the completion of this chapter, the reader will be able to:**

- discuss the three major volitional qualities: personal efficacy, values, and interests
- describe assessment indicators for each quality
- document objective and subjective assessment findings
- define key terms that may be used in this section of the psychiatric mental status examination

# HOW DO YOU ASSESS VOLITION?

Volition is the ability to use one's will. It is about making conscious decisions and acting on those decisions. In contrast, motivation is about the desire to do something, while volition is doing something about it. Without volition, a person is unable to engage in activities and relationships. Volition is also a factor in a person's capability to resist impulses. For example, volition may be impaired in people with anorexia nervosa, substance abuse, addiction to substances, and those who engage in other deliberate self-harm activities.

   Volition is a result of three inherent qualities: personal efficacy, values, and interests. Personal efficacy is related to an individual's views on whether they believe they have the skills and abilities to be successful. Values refer to the person's convictions and obligations to act in a certain way. Interests are about feeling attracted to performing an activity or behaviour. The stronger your belief is that you have the skills to make a difference—or how important it is to you to make a difference in an area of interest—the greater the likelihood that you will decide to actively decide to engage in an activity and will actually engage in that activity.

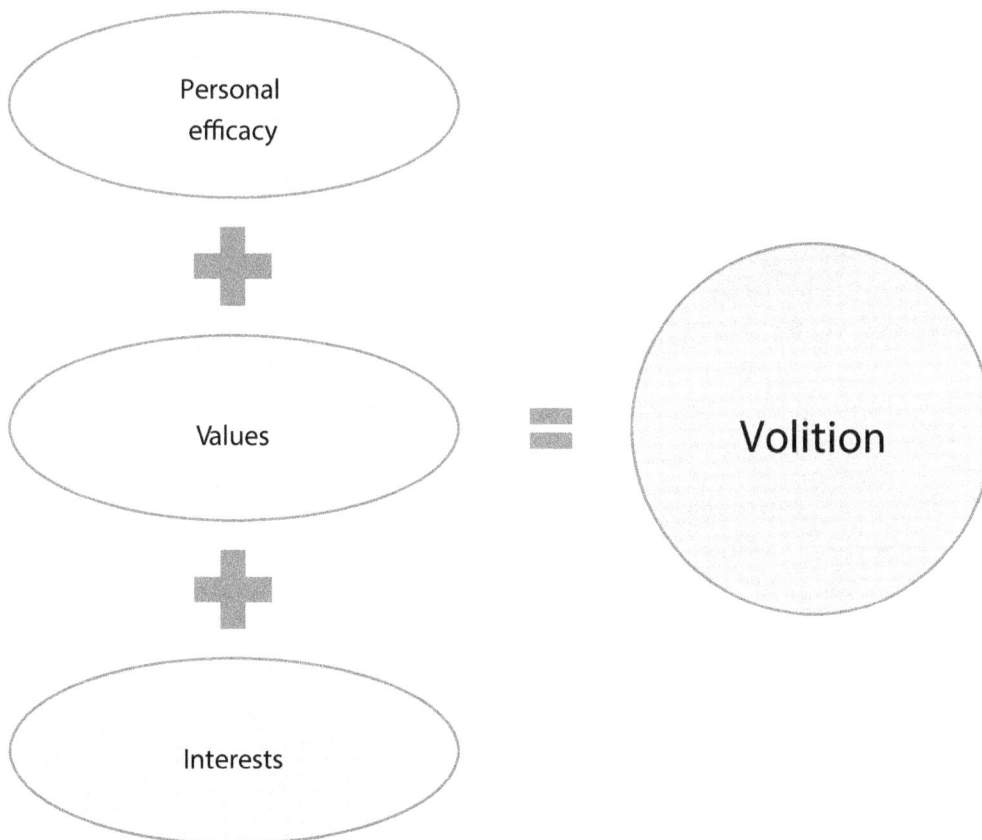

**Figure 12.1:** Volitional Qualities

Information about volition can be gathered by asking questions directly related to an individual's interests, values, and view of their own capabilities (strengths and weaknesses). Box 12.1 provides sample questions that may be used to explore volition. A clinician can also gather information from the client's psychiatric history. For example, questions related to how long the person has been employed, how long they have been in a relationship, and if they have a hobby and how they are able to stay engaged with this activity can yield information about personal efficacy, values, and interests.

## BOX 12.1: EXPLORING VOLITION

The following questions can be used to start a discussion that will allow you to delve deeper and explore volition:

- How would you describe yourself?
- When you start a project, how confident are you that you will finish it?
- What do you think is the likelihood that the treatment will reduce your symptoms? (Explore the reasons behind the client's answer.)
- What else have you tried to help with your symptoms? How long did you try this? What were the reasons you started, continued, or stopped?
- How would you describe your level of self-esteem? (Explore the reasons behind the client's answer.)
- What are your interests? Are there causes or hobbies that are important to you?
- What are your three important values? How are these demonstrated in your life? (Explore the reasons behind the client's answer.)
- What is your goal? What do you think is the likelihood of you achieving this goal? (Explore the reasons behind the client's answer.)

As with insight, volition also makes a significant impact on a clinician's ability to develop a therapeutic relationship; therefore, it is important to document findings that will help other team members effectively engage with the client and develop realistic treatment plans. Box 12.2 provides examples of how volition findings can be documented.

## BOX 12.2: DOCUMENTING VOLITION FINDINGS

### Norma

Norma describes being involved with several of her children's activities. She is president of the school parent council and is the treasurer for the local soccer club. Norma tells you that if you want something done, you should ask a busy person. She reports that once she sets her mind to something, it will get done.

**Ken**

Ken is a very driven nursing student. He is goal-directed and works hard to accomplish his goals in what he describes "as a reasonable time frame." He is trying to take this approach to treating his depression; however, he is finding it difficult to muster the energy to complete his daily cognitive exercises. He wishes that the pills would work faster.

## SPECIAL CONSIDERATIONS

The findings of the volition assessment will help the clinician to engage in treatment planning. Exploring what is important to the client and what they think their chances of success will be is an opportunity for the clinician to determine the client's degree of hopefulness.

## CHAPTER GLOSSARY TERMS

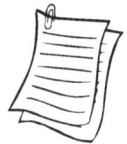

**directedness:** The ability to focus energy toward achieving goals.
**drive:** The ability to "carry on" or move forward toward goals.
**motivation:** The reasons one has to act.
**volition:** The ability to make a choice and act on it.
**willpower:** The determination to achieve.

## ACTIVITY: WHAT IS EXPECTED VERSUS UNEXPECTED?

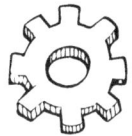

Complete table 12.1 and compare expected findings to common variations and unexpected findings for the three qualities of volition.

**Table 12.1:** Volition—Expected Findings, Common Variations, and Unexpected Findings

| Assessment area | Expected findings | Common variations | Unexpected findings/ further assessment required |
|---|---|---|---|
| *Sense of personal self-efficacy* | | | |

*continued*

| | | | |
|---|---|---|---|
| *Values* | | | |
| *Interests* | | | |

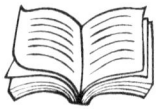

## STUDY QUESTIONS

1. Identify two questions that can be asked to explore each of the qualities of volition.

   _____
   _____
   _____
   _____
   _____
   _____
   _____
   _____
   _____
   _____

2. Why is it important to document the assessment findings for volition?

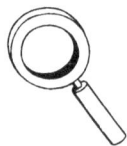

   _____
   _____
   _____
   _____

## CASE STUDY

Jaxxon is a heavy-duty equipment operator. He has come to the mental health clinic at the insistence of his wife because she finds him increasingly irritable and has threatened to leave if he doesn't see someone. Over the past couple of months, Jaxxon has felt unusually tired and has had increasingly greater difficulty concentrating at work. Although he has frequent disagreements at work, he is not worried about losing his job; however, he has started to eat lunch alone because there are so many annoying people that he just doesn't want to deal with. This is very different than his usual jovial disposition. During the interview, Jaxxon sits with his hands folded in his lap, eyes cast downward, and has a low monotone voice. He answers questions that are asked of him, but takes one to two minutes before he responds. When asked how he would describe his mood, he responds by saying, "What mood? I feel nothing." When asked what that means, he says, "I just feel numb. I have felt numb for the last month."

Jaxxon is deeply committed to his wife and needs to try something because she is so upset. He has been hospitalized for bipolar disorder in the past, but he tells you that this time feels different. He was given medication before, but it never really helped. This illness just needed to run its course.

## Case Study Question

Using the information provided in the case study, complete table 12.2 by identifying what information is provided for each of the volitional qualities.

**Table 12.2:** What Information Is Provided about Volition

| Assessment area | Information provided within the case study |
| --- | --- |
| *Sense of personal self-efficacy* | |
| *Values* | |
| *Interests* | |

# CHAPTER 13

## Physical Functioning

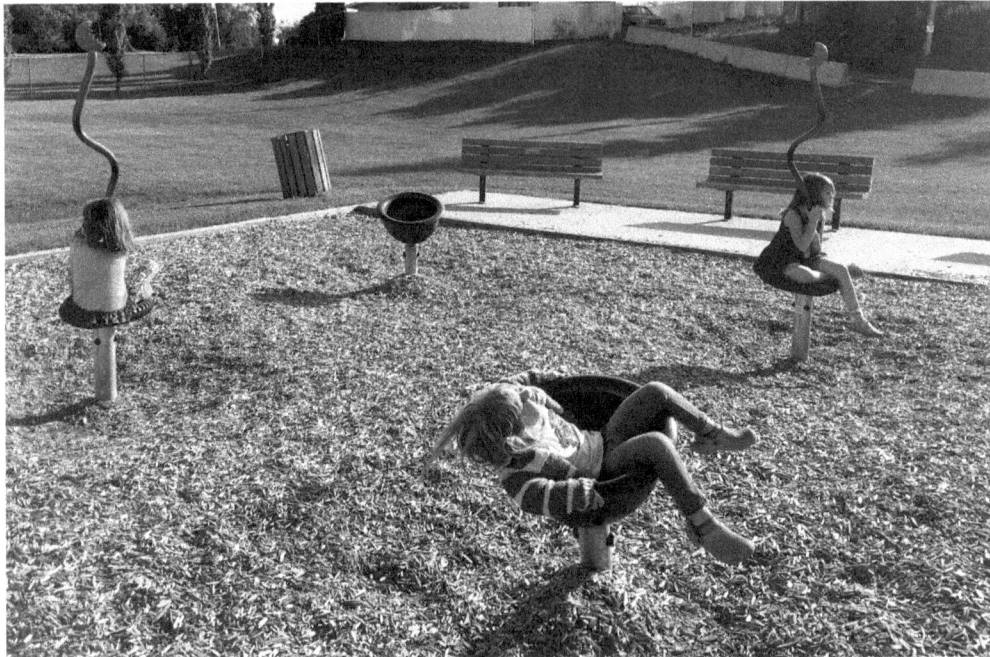

**Photo 13.1:** Mind and Body

> The secret of health for both mind and body is not to mourn for the past, not
> to worry about the future, or not to anticipate troubles, but to live the present
> moment wisely and earnestly.
> —*Siddartha Guatama Buddha*

## LEARNING OBJECTIVES

**At the completion of this chapter, the reader will be able to:**

- describe assessment indicators for physical functioning
- document objective and subjective assessment findings
- define key terms that may be used in this section of the psychiatric mental
  status examination

# PHYSICAL FUNCTIONING: DOES IT REALLY MATTER?

Alterations in physical functioning can affect many of the other areas of the mental status exam. People with psychiatric disorders have high rates of physical health problems including diabetes, cancer, and hypertension. There are also significant correlations between medical conditions and the experience of psychiatric symptoms. This includes depressed mood with hypothyroidism, anxiety with fluctuations in blood sugars, anxiety with chest pain, and psychosis with alterations in blood chemistry due to renal failure. As the psychiatric mental status examination is merely a snapshot of the client's presenting symptoms, knowing the client's general physical condition can help put the assessment data into perspective.

Your professional discipline will affect how you approach this section. Nurses and doctors tend to be very comfortable asking questions related to physical well-being, whereas social workers, family therapists, and art therapists may prefer to ask more general questions. This section is not meant to replace a full physical examination. In fact, when there are unexpected findings, further physical assessment is needed.

Asking general questions about health and physical well-being is what is required in this section. One approach is to begin with the question, "How is your general health?" The purpose of asking about physical health is that there are many mental disorders that affect our physical functioning. The most common changes are variations in sleep pattern, appetite, weight, nutritional status, and gastrointestinal functioning. The questions presented in box 13.1 can be used to start a discussion to assess physical functioning using a body systems approach. If the client has concerns with any of the questions asked of them, the clinician will need to further explore these concerns.

## BOX 13.1: EXPLORING PHYSICAL FUNCTIONING

The following questions can be asked to help explore a person's physical functioning:

- How have you been sleeping?
- Have there been any recent changes to your appetite or weight?
- Have you purged or vomited?
- Do you have any concerns about going to the bathroom?
- Have you had any recent concerns about your heart or breathing?
- Have you noticed any recent changes to your hair or skin?
- Do you have any concerns about your sexual functioning?
- How often do you get a cold or infection?
- Do you have any aches and pains?

While the clinician is documenting the session, they should note any change(s) or area(s) of concern. For example, if there has been a recent change in the client's weight, the documentation should include whether it was an increase or a decrease and the approximate amount of weight lost or gained. Changes in sleeping patterns should also be specifically recorded; for example, difficulty falling asleep, early morning awakening, or hypersomnia. Box 13.2 provides more specific examples of how to document physical functioning for the purposes of completing a psychiatric mental status exam.

## BOX 13.2: DOCUMENTING PHYSICAL INFORMATION

### Milo
Milo reports that she has no concerns regarding her physical functioning.

### Jon
Over the last two years, Jon has gained approximately 70 pounds; however, over the last two months his appetite has been very poor, but there has been no accompanying weight loss. He reports that he sleeps for about three hours a day. He can fall asleep, but then wakes up after an hour or two. Jon believes that if he could get some restful sleep, his other problems would resolve. Jon reports that he has Ménière's disease and uses self-prescribed herbal remedies for his arthritis. He believes that these diseases are currently under control.

## SPECIAL CONSIDERATIONS

Many diseases have cognitive, emotional, and behavioural symptoms. Any condition that has the potential to affect the client's mental state should be recorded; examples include temporal lobe epilepsy, asthma, liver failure, hypothyroidism, and multiple sclerosis. Collaboration with other members of the health care team is often beneficial in providing information when there are unexpected findings in this area.

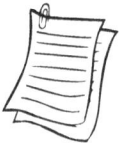

## CHAPTER GLOSSARY TERMS

**anorexia:** Loss of appetite or diminished food intake.

**cardiovascular system:** Pertains to parts of the body that circulate blood, including the heart, arteries, and veins.

**digestive system:** Pertains to parts of body that provide nutrition through mechanical and chemical processes, including the mouth, stomach, intestines, and elimination processes.

**endocrine system:** Pertains to the chemical communication system within the body; it includes hormones but excludes neurotransmitters.

**hyperphagia:** Excessive food intake; increased appetite.

**hypersomnia:** Excessive sleep.

**insomnia:** The inability to sleep satisfactorily, either quantitatively (the number of hours) or qualitatively (restless sleep).

**integumentary system:** Pertains to parts that cover the body, including skin, hair, and nails.

**lymphatic system:** Pertains to parts of the body that carry lymphatic fluid.

**musculoskeletal system:** Pertains to parts supporting and moving parts of the body, including the skeleton, tendons, and muscles.

**nervous system:** Pertains to collecting and processing information; it includes the brain, nerves, and neurotransmitters.

**reproductive system:** Pertains to creating another; it includes sexual functioning.

**respiratory system:** Pertains to moving air in and out of the body; it includes the lungs.

# ACTIVITY: WHAT BODY SYSTEM ARE YOU ASKING ABOUT?

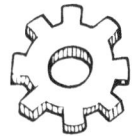

For each of the questions in table 13.1, identify what body system is being investigated.

**Table 13.1:** Investigating Physical Functioning

| Question | Corresponding body system |
|---|---|
| *How have you been sleeping?* | |
| *Have there been any recent changes to your appetite or weight?* | |
| *Do you have any concerns about going to the bathroom?* | |

*continued*

| | |
|---|---|
| *Have you had any recent concerns about your heart?* | |
| *Have you noticed any recent changes to your hair or skin?* | |
| *Do you have any concerns about your sexual functioning?* | |
| *How often do you get a cold or infection?* | |
| *Do you have any aches and pains?* | |

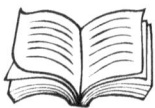

# STUDY QUESTIONS

1.  Identify two physical functioning alterations that can result in a person experiencing anxiety?

    _____
    _____
    _____
    _____

2.  If more information about physical functioning were necessary, where would you refer your client? Why?

    _____
    _____
    _____

_____

_____


**3.** Why is physical functioning included in a psychiatric mental status examination?

_____

_____

_____

_____


# CASE STUDY

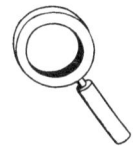

Jules is a 19-year-old female who attends university and lives with her parents. Her parents describe her as always being very particular about her food, but say that this seems to have "gotten out of hand" over the last two months. Jules has never been overweight. Over the last two months, Jules has withdrawn and has lost 25 pounds.

Jules has always done well in school. She describes herself as a perfectionist. She likes to be at the top of her class. Two months ago, she failed a pathophysiology exam. She has never failed at anything before. At that time, she started to miss the occasional meal so she could study. Because her time was so precious, she started to eat only fruit and fries, avoiding meat and any other carbohydrates. Jules's friends started to tease her about how big her clothes were getting and began to say that she really needed to have a burger with the fries. When this pattern started, she began to eat only in private and stopped socializing with her friends.

At home, she complained about feeling cold all the time and would often wear a sweater and a coat. It was obvious to her parents that she wasn't eating properly. Jules was insistent that there weren't any issues with her eating and nothing was wrong. Her parents made an appointment at the primary care centre because they knew something was wrong and she wouldn't talk to them about her troubles.

## Case Study Questions


**1.** Imagine that you are a member of the staff at the primary care centre. What is the first question that you should ask?

_____

_____

_____

_____

2.  What are three strategies you would use to build a therapeutic relationship with Jules?

    _____

    _____

    _____

    _____

3.  After assessing Jules's physical functioning, what area of the mental status exam should be assessed next? Why?

    _____

    _____

    _____

    _____

# CHAPTER 14

## Putting It All Together

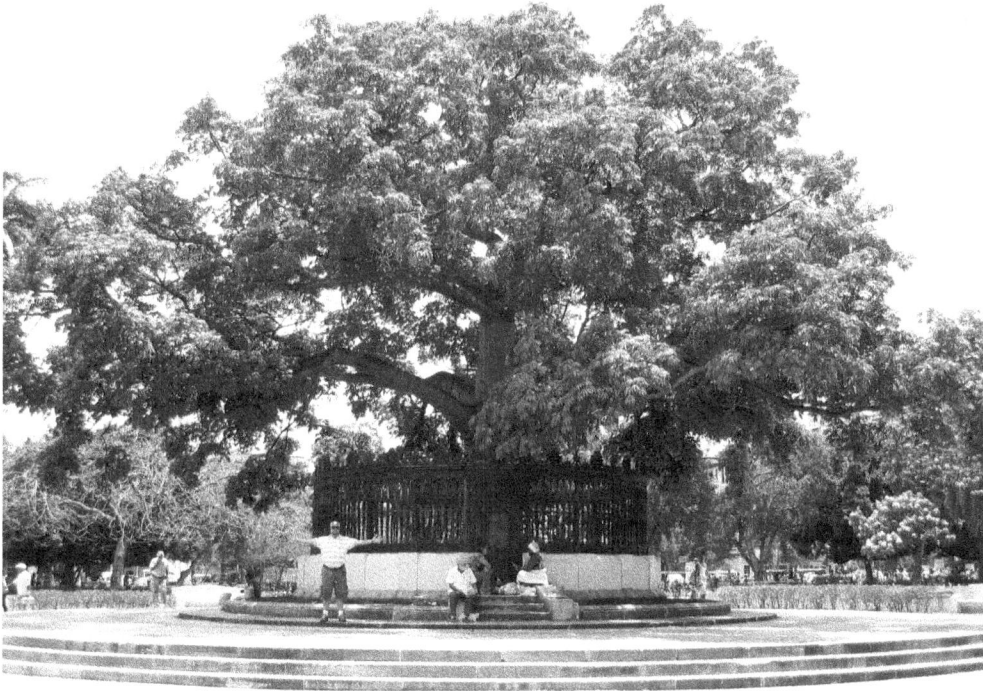

**Photo 14.1:** And Then There Was One

> Anyone who has never made a mistake has never tried anything new.
> —*Albert Einstein*

## LEARNING OBJECTIVES

**At the completion of this chapter, the reader will be able to:**

- discuss all 11 sections of the psychiatric mental status examination
- describe means of collecting assessment data in each of the areas of the mental status examination
- document a complete mental status examination

# NOW WHAT?

There are 11 different sections of the psychiatric mental status examination. There is no one "correct" way to complete this assessment. How you complete the assessment will depend on your discipline and your experience conducting the mental status exam. Many novice clinicians follow the order presented on the exam, but over time every clinician develops their own "flow" in completing the assessment. When conducting assessments, clinicians are encouraged to try different approaches and use different questions to fully assess each of the areas. It is important to remember that clinicians should first document what is expected, what is a common variation, and what is unexpected as the basis for the client evaluations. Any unexpected findings will need further exploration.

As you start to think about how you will conduct your own mental status examinations, first consider how you will collect the information. Table 14.1 presents the 11 sections of the mental status exam and identifies how information for each section is collected.

**Table 14.1:** Collecting Mental Status Information

| Section of mental status examination | Method of data collection | |
| --- | --- | --- |
| | Observation | Discussion and inquiry |
| *General description* | X | |
| *Emotional state* | X | X |
| *Speech* | X | |
| *Thought processes* | X | |
| *Thought content* | | X |
| *Risk assessment* | | X |
| *Perception* | X | X |

| | | |
|---|---|---|
| *Cognitive state* | X | X |
| *Insight* | X | X |
| *Volition* | X | X |
| *Physical functioning* | X | X |

After reflecting on the general sections of the mental status exam, use the following activity to think about the categories within each of the major sections. Next, read the case study and identify all the components of the mental status exam that are described.

# ACTIVITY: COLLECTING INFORMATION ON MENTAL STATUS EXAMINATION SECTION CATEGORIES

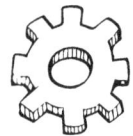

In table 14.2, identify how data is collected for the identified section categories of the mental status examination. What questions would you ask to gather more information?

**Table 14.2:** Collecting Information on Mental Status Exam Section Categories

| Section of mental status examination | Method of data collection | |
|---|---|---|
| | Observation:<br>What do you need to observe? | Discussion and inquiry:<br>What questions would you ask to gather more information? |
| *Appearance* | | |
| *Behaviour* | | |
| *Attitude* | | |

*continued*

| | | |
|---|---|---|
| *Mood* | | |
| *Affect* | | |
| *Volume of speech* | | |
| *Rate of speech* | | |
| *Quality of speech* | | |
| *Clarity of speech* | | |
| *Comprehension of speech* | | |
| *Rate of thought processes* | | |
| *Flow of thought processes* | | |
| *Form of thought processes* | | |
| *Delusions* | | |
| *Command hallucinations* | | |
| *Depersonalization* | | |

| | | |
|---|---|---|
| **Misidentification** | | |
| **Abstract thinking** | | |
| **Judgment** | | |
| **Intellectual ability** | | |
| **General information** | | |
| **Memory** | | |
| **Orientation** | | |
| **Concentration and attention** | | |
| **Consciousness** | | |
| **Personal efficacy** | | |
| **Values** | | |
| **Interests** | | |

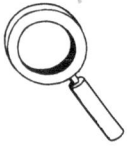

# CASE STUDY

A middle-aged man enters the clinic. He is breathing a little erratically and somewhat quickly. You notice that he is wearing a women's light raincoat although it is a beautiful day outside. His hair is dishevelled and he has five o'clock shadow. He seems to be in average physical condition because you notice his stomach clearly when he takes off his coat. He nervously accepts your offer to sit. As he sits down, you notice that his socks do not match and that his shoes need polishing. He does not seem comfortable in the chair because he continues to shift around.

He makes eye contact with you but never for very long. His eyes move around and appear to be scanning your office. You ask him how you can be of help. His conversation moves like his eyes. He begins to speak very quickly: "Thanks so much for seeing me. I really appreciate it." He thanks you several times again. "I don't know where to begin," he says. You have difficulty following his train of thought and several times you ask questions to try to make sense of what he is saying. "Well, you see, it's my wife, and my job, well, it's not good, but it's not dead yet, but my wife…." His voice rises as he speaks, then he becomes quiet and mumbles to himself.

"I feel agitated all the time. I can't ever relax. I feel like I am just wound up so tightly right now," he shares with you. As the interview progresses, he seems to settle down a bit, but he shares that he is usually uptight. "I can't get the business out of my mind," he says. "It is so close to doing great. Do you know anything about the communications field?" he asks you. "This is so big! It's going to revolutionize the communications industry." You are silent, but he continues, "I am starting on the ground floor of an emerging market that will transform how we all think about communication! My wife just doesn't see it that way." He shares his story of how the business started and how he met his wife: "I remember when I first met her just after college. I couldn't understand what she saw in me, but I guess I tricked her into marrying me. I was never very attractive or athletic and the girls were never lining up to see me, but she really liked me."

You learn that he has owned a small business for two years, but is about to declare bankruptcy. His wife left him two weeks ago and he has been staying at the YMCA since she left. He lost his jacket and borrowed his secretary's raincoat upon leaving work because he heard it was going to rain. He asks if you can prescribe him some medication. He shares that he has an important meeting to make at 4:00 p.m., so he needs to be going. "You're a really great listener," he says on his way out. "I'll see you next time."

## Case Study Question

Complete a psychiatric mental status examination for the client described in the case study. Make sure to cover all 11 areas. Use the client's own words to back up your statements.

# CHAPTER 15

## What Do You Do with a Completed Psychiatric Mental Status Examination?

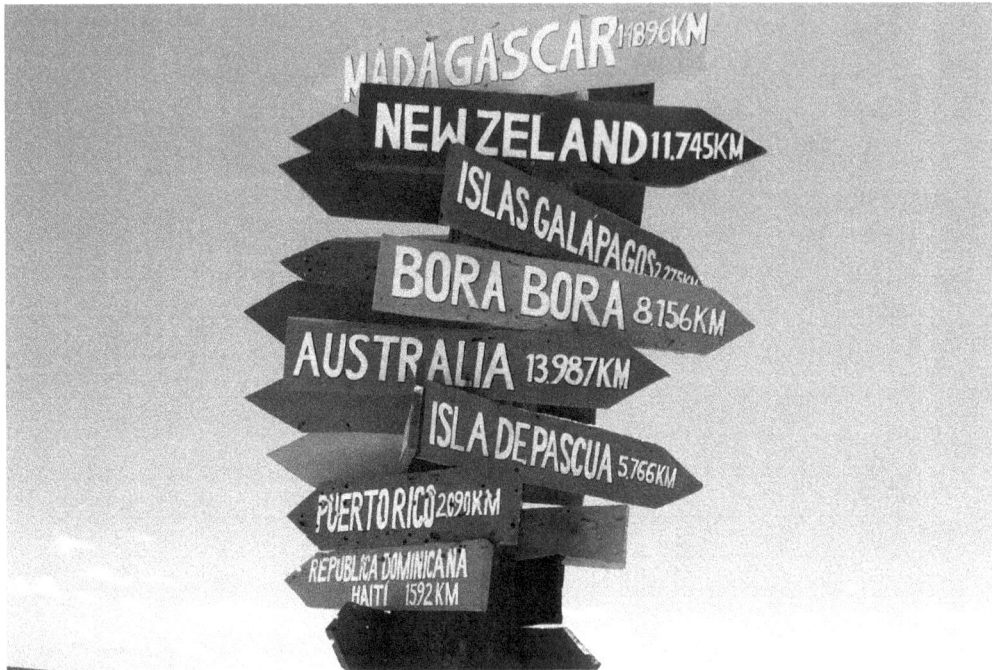

**Photo 15.1:** Deciding Where to Go Next

We are where we are, however we got here. What matters is where we go next.
—*Isaac Marion*

## LEARNING OBJECTIVES

**At the completion of this chapter, the reader will be able to:**

- identify what to do with a completed mental status examination
- discuss priority areas to communicate with other team members

# NEXT STEPS

Once the psychiatric mental status assessment has been completed, it needs to be compared to and combined with information gathered from the biopsychosocial and spiritual history, and auxiliary information from other sources (friends or family of the client, psychological investigations, and, if indicated, medical examinations). This is done to determine the reliability of the information that has been obtained. Factors that affect reliability include the client's age, intellectual abilities, motivation, and the presence of psychotic or neurocognitive symptoms.

The results are then communicated to other members of the treatment team, including the client. This information forms the foundation for determining a treatment plan and most responsible diagnosis, and determining prognosis. The assessment results related to risk are the most essential to communicate to other team members and should be highlighted in your documentation. You will then collaboratively developed strategies to reduce changeable risk factors (see box 15.1).

## BOX 15.1: CHANGEABLE RISK FACTORS

- access to lethality
- addictions
- isolation
- lack of capacity within support systems
- lack of responsiveness to treatment
- no access to health care
- response to stress
- untreated or worsening mental health disorder

# EXAMPLE OF A PSYCHIATRIC MENTAL STATUS EXAMINATION

There are many ways to complete a mental status examination. The following is an example of how a completed mental status examination may be written. Imagine that you are working in the emergency department of your local hospital.

## Background

Mr. Jack Spade is a 29-year-old male who arrived from home via ambulance at 9:00 p.m. He was dressed in cotton pajamas. Mr. Spade had been discharged from the surgical unit seven days earlier after the wound on his coccyx was debrided. He had called the ambulance after he had fallen in the bathroom, hitting his head on the sink, which resulted in a four-centimetre cut above his eyebrow.

## Mental Status

Mr. Spade is a 29-year-old male who was interviewed in the emergency department shortly after he received stiches for a cut above his right eyebrow. He was wearing blood-stained pajamas. He lay near motionless in bed during the entire interview. Although he was soft-spoken, he was articulate, and volunteered information when he thought he had additional relevant information to share. Mr. Spade described his mood as depressed and reported that he has been on antidepressants for nearly two years. Over the course of the last two months, his mood has been lower, he has lost nearly 20 pounds, and he has had a very difficult time falling asleep although he reports feeling very tired. The affect demonstrated was consistent with his mood and topic of conversation. Rate of thought was slow; however, there was purposeful connectedness and organization to his thoughts.

He reported that since his surgery, he has had a hard time facing people and doesn't want to go out of the house because he is embarrassed. When specifically asked about suicide, he reported that he frequently thinks that his life may not be worth living. He stated that his father hung himself when Jack was nine years old. The suicide came just after his father was accused of sexually molesting his sons. Jack stated that he wouldn't hang himself, like his dad did, as this was just one more way that he abused them—he hung himself in the house to be sure that Jack or one of his brothers found him. Jack is an avid hunter and has ready access to firearms and ammunition. He stated that he would only need one shot and would do it in a place where no one would find him. He denied plans to kill himself within the next two weeks. He stated that he still needed to look after a few things before he would be ready to "meet his maker." Occasionally, Jack described feeling like his father was touching his body again. This has become a daily occurrence since his surgery. He stated that this "freaks him out. Even though I know he's not there."

Mr. Spade was able to accurately identify the date and the location of the interview. He had a broad general information fund. Although he was not able to recall exactly what happened just before he fell, he was able to extrapolate a logical explanation for the injury. When asked why he thought the last two months had been difficult for him, he clearly stated that he was having a hard time coping with losing his job, and that he had started to have flashbacks since the surgery.

He described feeling very tired and extremely frustrated because he thought he had put all "this stuff" with this father behind him and now he needs to deal with it again. He is not sure he has the strength to do that.

## STUDY QUESTIONS

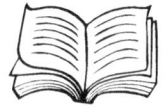

1.  What piece of information is most important to share with the team members? Why?

_____

_____

_____

_____

2.  What are Mr. Spade's changeable risk factors?

_____

_____

_____

_____

_____

3.  Mr. Spade is ready for discharge. What are your next steps?

_____

_____

_____

_____

_____

_____

_____

_____

_____

_____

# Activity Answers

Potential answers are provided below for the activities included in chapters 5, 6, 7, and 11.

## CHAPTER 5: SPEECH

### Speech Linkage with Other Areas of the Mental Status Examination Answers

- Speech is an important part of language development. **True**
- It is normal for a child of two years of age to say fewer than 50 words and to not use any two-word combinations (e.g., "more drink," "Mommy gone," "truck go"). **False**
- Difficulty answering questions may be related to biological factors. **True**
- Difficulty sequencing words in sentences is related to speech development. **True**
- An expressive language delay results in difficulty getting across ideas and thoughts. **True**
- A receptive language delay results in difficulty understanding instructions and questions. **True**
- Language difficulties can result in trouble interacting with peers. **True**
- Language difficulties can result in poor working memory. **True**
- Language difficulties can result in poor attention and concentration. **True**
- Fun play-based activities or games can be used to help motivate a child to learn. **True**

## CHAPTER 6: THOUGHT PROCESSES

**Table 6.1:** Alphabet Soup Puzzle Answer

|   |   | H | A | L | L | U | C | I | N | A | T | E |   |
|---|---|---|---|---|---|---|---|---|---|---|---|---|---|
| O | R | G | A | N | I | Z | E |   |   |   |   |   |   |
|   |   |   |   |   | P | H | O | B | I | A |   |   |   |
|   |   |   | D | R | A | M | A | T | I | C |   |   |   |
|   |   |   |   |   | A | P | A | T | H | Y |   |   |   |
|   |   |   | A | G | I | T | A | T | E | D |   |   |   |
|   |   |   |   | I | N | Q | U | I | R | E |   |   |   |

| | | | P | L | A | C | E | | | | | |
|---|---|---|---|---|---|---|---|---|---|---|---|---|
| | | | | D | Y | S | T | O | N | I | C | |
| P | E | R | P | L | E | X | E | D | | | | |
| | | | | | W | I | T | H | D | R | A | W |
| | | | B | E | H | A | V | I | O | U | R | |
| | | | | H | Y | P | E | R | | | | |
| I | N | C | O | N | G | R | U | E | N | T | | |
| | | | | O | B | S | E | S | S | | | |
| | | | D | E | L | I | R | I | U | M | | |
| | | | | N | E | G | L | E | C | T | | |
| | L | A | B | I | L | E | | | | | | |
| | | | | J | U | D | G | M | E | N | T | |
| | F | R | A | N | K | | | | | | | |
| | | | | I | L | L | U | S | I | O | N | |
| | | F | I | D | G | E | T | | | | | |
| | | F | E | A | R | F | U | L | | | | |
| | | | D | E | S | P | A | I | R | | | |
| | | | | E | V | A | S | I | V | E | | |
| | | | A | M | B | I | V | A | L | E | N | T |

# CHAPTER 7: THOUGHT CONTENT

**Table 7.1:** Developmental Refresher Answers

| Age | Erikson | Piaget | Developmental tasks | Coping skills |
|---|---|---|---|---|
| *Infancy* *(0–1 year)* | Basic trust versus mistrust | Sensorimotor (birth–2 years) | · learn to coordinate sensory experience and motor behaviour<br>· treatment by caregivers creates trust in a good world<br>· hope<br>· appreciation of interdependence and relatedness | · crying<br>· kicking<br>· motor activity—gratification or tension reduction |

*continued*

| Age | Erikson | Piaget | Developmental tasks | Coping skills |
|---|---|---|---|---|
| **Early childhood (2–3 years)** | Autonomy versus shame | Preoperational (2–7 years) | · egocentrism<br>· child is either allowed to make independent decisions or is made to feel ashamed/full of doubt about own decisions<br>· will<br>· acceptance of the cycle of life, from integration to disintegration<br>· questioning through play<br>· assertion of independence | · repetitive play<br>· protest<br>· fantasy<br>· comfort<br>· time out<br>· experimentation<br>· restricting environment |
| **Play age (4–5 years)** | Initiative versus guilt | Preoperational (2–7 years) | · child either develops own purpose/direction or is made to feel guilty by overly controlling caregivers<br>· understands right from wrong<br>· magical thinking<br>· purpose<br>· humour, empathy, resilience<br>· independent activity<br>· role and identity in family<br>· maintain and protect body integrity | · routines<br>· ritualized activity<br>· hiding |
| **School age (6–11 years)** | Industry versus inferiority | Concrete operational (7–11 years) | · learn to logically reason about objects<br>· can make inferences from conversations<br>· child either feels compe-tent working with others or inferior<br>· competence<br>· humility, acceptance of the course of one's life and unfulfilled hopes<br>· peer relationships<br>· acceptance | · humour<br>· problem solving<br>· withdrawal<br>· aggression<br>· control of behaviour<br>· confide in friends<br>· selects what they will tell parents |

| Age | Erikson | Piaget | Developmental tasks | Coping skills |
|-----|---------|--------|---------------------|---------------|
| **Adolescence** **(12–19 years)** | Identity versus confusion | Formal operational (adolescent to adult) | · reasoning more abstract and logical<br>· adolescent either grasps sense of identity or becomes confused about possible future roles as adult<br>· fidelity<br>· sense of complexity of life, and merging of sensory, logical, and aesthetic perception<br>· self-consciousness<br>· competitive | · denial<br>· intellectualization<br>· conformity<br>· emotional control<br>· motor activity<br>· withdrawal<br>· solicit opinions of peers |
| **Early adulthood** **(20–25 years)** | Intimacy versus isolation | Formal operational (adolescent to adult) | · either forming deep/intimate relationships with others or becoming socially isolated<br>· love<br>· sense of complexity of relationships, value of tenderness and loving freely | · coping mechanisms<br>· withdrawal |
| **Adulthood** **(26–64 years)** | Generativity versus stagnation | Formal operational (adolescent to adult) | · either determining what to leave behind for future generations or failing to grasp a sense of meaning in life<br>· caring for others, empathy and concern | · coping mechanisms<br>· withdrawal |
| **Old age** **(65 years to death)** | Integrity versus despair | Formal operational (adolescent to adult) | · either feeling that life was worthwhile or feeling despair about one's life and fearing death<br>· wisdom<br>· existential identity, a sense of integrity strong enough to withstand physical disintegration | · coping mechanisms<br>· withdrawal |

# CHAPTER 11: INSIGHT

## Insight Matching Exercise Answers

4   affect
2   general observations
11  insight
9   judgment
8   memory
5   mood
10  orientation
7   perceptions
1   sensorium
3   speech characteristics
6   thinking

# Glossary

**abstract thinking:** The ability to generalize thinking and to form ideas that are part of an instance or material objects, but are not concrete.

**abusive:** Language that is extremely derogatory.

**accelerated:** Tempo of speech is rapid, giving the impression that a client feels hurried and pushed.

**affect:** The emotional feeling or tone attached to an object, idea, or thought. This includes inner feelings and their external manifestations.

**affective interaction:** Behaviour during an interview that is emotionally charged.

**aggressive:** Forceful behaviour, whether verbal or physical. It is the motor counterpart to the affect of anger or hostility.

**agitation:** Restless, volatile, or erratic emotional behaviour accompanied by a great deal of motor restlessness and often anxiety.

**akinesia:** A lack of physical movement.

**aloof:** Distant; emotionally uninvolved.

**ambivalent:** The presence of strong, simultaneously contrasting feelings; the ability to hold simultaneously opposite feelings.

**amnesia:** A disturbance in memory manifested by partial or total inability to recall past experiences.

**angry:** Strong feelings of annoyance or hostility.

**animated:** Facial expression is suitably responsive to the present stimulus or situation. This includes positive responses such as smiling, brightness, and spontaneity.

**anorexia:** Loss of appetite or diminished food intake.

**anxiety:** An unpleasurable affect consisting of physical changes and a subjective feeling of fear. In contrast to normal fear, the danger or threat in anxiety is unreal. The subjective feeling is an uncomfortable dread of impending danger, accompanied by an overwhelming awareness of being powerless, an inability to perceive the unreality of the threat, a prolonged feeling of tension, and an exhaustive readiness for the expected danger.

**apathetic:** Feeling no interest.

**apathy:** Lack of interest or emotional involvement in one's surroundings.

**apprehensive:** Mood is characterized by feelings of fear, uncertainty, insecurity, and anxiety; a sense of being threatened.

**appropriate:** Suitable for the ensuing and present activity or environment.

**appropriate behaviour:** Behaviour is suited to the requirements of the prevailing situation.

**appropriate clothing:** Clothing worn is suitable for the ensuing activity or environment.

**assaultive:** Physically aggressive and threatening; striking out at others.

**attention:** The aspect of consciousness that relates to the amount of effort exerted in focusing on certain aspects of an experience. It is sometimes used interchangeably with *concentration*.

**auditory hallucination:** A sound that does not have a concrete, external stimulus. For some people who hear voices, the voices will be clear, whereas for others they may sound like a constant mumbling in the background. Some people hear only one voice, but others may hear a number of different voices at the same time.

**automatic obedience:** A pathological degree of compliance with the instructions of the examiner.

**awareness:** Knowing that something exists.

**belligerent:** Combative, quarrelsome, argumentative, hostile, defiant.

**bizarre:** Unconventional, characterized by strange or eccentric mannerisms, dress, ideas or acts.

**blocking:** Intellectual processes that are characterized by sudden stoppages in the sequential flow of thought and speech.

**blunted:** Diminution of affect; lacking the normal range of responsiveness of mood.

**bored:** Mild degree of emotional detachment indicated by little interest being shown in the conversation or activity, and by signs of weariness and indifference to the activity.

**cardiovascular system:** Pertains to parts of the body that circulate blood, including the heart, arteries, and veins.

**cataleptic:** Condition in which the person maintains the body position into which they are placed.

**catastrophic anxiety:** The extreme and overwhelming anxiety that is felt when a client with an organic brain syndrome becomes aware of the defects in his mentation.

**changeable:** Emotionally labile; frequently changing moods.

**change pattern:** The rate of change of emotional expression. It is characterized as stable (normal rate of change) or labile (rapid change in emotional expression without external stimuli).

**circumstantial:** Talking around the point but never getting to it.

**clang speech:** Improper use of words based on sound of the words; similar to punning and rhyming, which is music-like speech.

**clarity:** Describes whether speech is understandable or if there is slurring, mumbling, or stuttering.

**clear:** Speech that follows an orderly, grammatical pattern; words are appropriately used and easily understood.

**clouding of consciousness:** A disturbance of consciousness characterized by unclear sensory perceptions due to diminished alertness and apparent inability to concentrate.

**cognition:** The mental process of knowing, thinking, and becoming aware.

**command hallucination:** A unique kind of auditory hallucination in which a voice that is giving instructions to a person does not have a concrete, external stimulus.

**complaintive:** Given to complaining, blaming, or being overly critical.

**compulsions:** Involuntary, uncontrollable, repetitive behavioural acts or rituals that the client feels compelled to carry out because of a feeling of anxiety.

**compulsive movements:** The result of an irresistible urge to perform a certain act. For example, the uncontrollable need to continually wash one's hands.

**confabulation:** Retrospective falsification of memory.

**confusion:** Diminished awareness, alertness, and impaired sensorium; difficulty grasping a situation, accompanied by disorientation with regard to time, place, and person.

**congruent:** Appropriate response or expression to the presence of stimuli or situation.

**consciousness:** The level of awareness and degree of alertness.

**coordinated:** Movements exhibit a normal degree of flexibility and harmony with no sign of impaired motor control.

**decreased interest:** Intellectual behaviour that shows signs of diminishing awareness of, response to, or concern about others, employment, activities, and surroundings; this is indicative of varying degrees of recession into a state of mental and emotional detachment.

**defensive:** Tendency to rationalize or make excuses.

**delirium:** A disturbance in the state of consciousness stemming from an organic reaction characterized by restlessness, confusion, disorientation, bewilderment, agitation, and affective lability.

**delusions:** Beliefs that are not true to fact, cannot be corrected by an appeal to reason of the individual, and are out of harmony with their educational and cultural background.

**delusions of control:** False beliefs that one is being manipulated by others.

**delusions of grandeur:** False beliefs consisting of an exaggerated concept of one's own importance.

**delusions of infidelity:** False beliefs that one's lover is unfaithful.

**delusions of reference:** False beliefs that the behaviour of others refers to oneself.

**delusions of self-accusation:** False feelings of remorse or guilt.

**demanding:** Persistently requiring attention.

**dementia:** An older term used to indicate organic loss of mental functioning. *Major neurocognitive disorder* is the current diagnostic term.

**denial:** Erroneously believing that one's problem, difficulty, or illness is not present.

**dependent:** Tendency to look to others for emotional support, to require constant reassurance and direction, and to cling.

**depth:** The level of complexity and extent of feelings and thoughts.

**despair:** Utter abandonment of hope.

**digestive system:** pertains to parts of body that provide nutrition through mechanical and chemical processes, including the mouth, stomach, intestines, and elimination processes.

**directedness:** The ability to focus energy toward achieving goals.

**drive:** The ability to "carry on" or move forward toward goals.

**duration:** The persistence of the mood, measured in hours, days, weeks, months, or even years.

**dysphoric:** A general feeling of melancholy.

**dystonic:** A motor disturbance usually observed as a side effect of phenothiazine drugs and major tranquilizers that consists of uncoordinated and spasmodic movements of the body and limbs, such as arching of the back and twisting of the body and neck.

**echopraxia:** Imitation of another person's movements.

**ecstatic:** Ecstasy; an affect of intense rapture.

**elation:** A high degree of excitement and euphoria in which the client may be expansive, feel invulnerable, and claim that they have never felt better.

**emotional:** Speech that is heavily covered with affective tone.

**endocrine system:** Pertains to the chemical communication system within the body; it includes hormones but excludes neurotransmitters.

**euphoria:** An exaggerated sense of well-being inappropriate to the apparent events.

**euphoric:** A feeling of intense excitement and happiness.

**evasive:** Rationalizes behaviour, evades or disowns responsibility, and covers up.

**expressionless:** Face registers no specific emotion; appears blank, immobile, unresponsive, and emotionless.

**exultation:** Similar to *euphoria* and *elation* but to a greater degree; intense elation and feelings of grandeur.

**facial expression:** The positioning of one's facial muscles that is often used to convey a feeling.

**fatigued:** Face may be haggard or drawn, showing signs of stress, tension, exhaustion, tiredness, and defeat.

**fearful:** Expression reflecting apprehension, fright, tension, or strain.

**flat:** Similar to *blunted*, indicating an extreme degree of emotional detachment and a lack of normal emotional responsiveness characterized by complete lack of visible emotion and affect.

**flight of ideas:** Thought patterns consisting of a rapid succession of ideas with little or no visible connection; a tendency for the client to start talking on one subject, then rapidly switch to another subject, then another, with very little connection between topics.

**flirtatious:** Seductive and sexually playful.

**gait:** The manner in which a person walks.

**general description:** The overall appearance of the client, including posture, dress, personal care, hygiene, weight, bearing, movement, and facial expression.

**gesture:** The movement of a body part to convey an idea or a feeling.

**grieving:** The alteration in mood or affect that consists of sadness appropriate to a real loss.

**grimacing:** Expression consisting of voluntary or involuntary frowning, scowling, or contorted facial movements reflecting disgust, disapproval, and so on.

**grooming:** The activity of tending to one's appearance and hygiene.

**guilt:** Affect associated with self-reproach and the need for punishment.

**gustatory hallucination:** A taste that does not have a concrete external stimulus.

**hallucinations:** Sensory perceptions that do not have a concrete external stimulus.

**hesitant:** Speech that is characterized by large pauses between words, as if indicating uncertainty.

**homicidal:** Intent to kill another.

**hypermnesia:** Exaggerated degree of retention and recall. It is observed sometimes in schizophrenia, manic drug intoxications, and hypnosis.

**hyperphagia:** Excessive food intake; increased appetite.

**hypersomnia:** Excessive sleep.

**hypochondriacal thoughts:** Occur when a client is morbidly concerned about their physical health or persistently complains of various physical ailments, though medical evidence will not support their claim.

**hysterical:** Behaviour that is marked by excitable, emotional outbursts.

**ideas of influence:** Feelings that one is capable of influencing the behaviour of others or situations through one's thoughts or desires; closely related to grandiose delusions.

**ideas of reference:** Misinterpretation of incidents and events in the outside world as having a direct, personal significance, or reference to oneself.

**illogical:** Speech that lacks coherence, is disorganized and unintelligible, and may consist of words and phrases that are garbled, vague, and nonsensical, including neologisms and word salad. The speech pattern may be broken down by irregular interruptions, halting, and blocking.

**illusions:** Misinterpretations of actual sensory stimuli. Illusions should be carefully distinguished from hallucinations. Illusions may occur in any sensory modality.

**inattentive:** Indifferent and lacks interest.

**incongruent:** Inappropriate response or expression to the presence of stimuli or situation.

**indifference:** Lacks interest in and concern about the conversation.

**initiates:** Spontaneously begins a conversation in response.

**insecurity:** Feelings of helplessness and inadequacy in the face of anxiety about one's place, future, and goals.

**insight:** Awareness and understanding of one's illness and the symptoms of illness, with or without an awareness of their cause and result.

**insomnia:** The inability to sleep satisfactorily, either quantitatively (the number of hours) or qualitatively (restless sleep).

**integumentary system:** Pertains to parts that cover the body, including skin, hair, and nails.

**intensity:** The strength of emotional expression. It is characterized as average, flat (complete lack of emotional expression), or blunted (reduced intensity of emotional expression).

**intent:** Level of determination.

**irrelevant:** Thoughts appear to be out of place and not normally associated with the topic at hand.

**irritable:** Short-tempered, easily angered or upset, and impatient, with a low frustration tolerance.

**jocular:** Playful, joking interaction.

**judgment:** The mental act of comparing or evaluating choices within the framework of a given set of values to select a course of action. Judgment is said to be intact if the course of action is consistent with reality.

**kinesthetic hallucination:** A sensation that a body part is moving without a concrete, external stimulus.

**labile:** Changeable, unstable.

**logical:** Speech follows an orderly grammatical pattern and is appropriately used and easy to understand.

**loud:** Greater volume than usual.

**lymphatic system:** Pertains to parts of the body that carry lymphatic fluid.

**mannerisms:** Are seen in most people, are not as persistent as stereotypes, and are more in keeping with the individual's personality. They are more frequently in evidence in people under some stress. Examples include shoulder shrugging, repeatedly clearing the throat, and blinking.

**melancholic:** A specific type of depressed affect characterized by insomnia and agitation, and sometimes paranoid ideas.

**mental status:** The organized recording of a psychiatric interview and examination in which the clinician's observations of the client's behaviour and replies to specific questions are carefully documented to give a picture of the client's general health, appearance, speech, form and content of thought, perceptual processes, state of consciousness, cognitive state, insight, and judgment.

**monotone:** Lack of normal modulation in tone.

**motivation:** The reasons one has to act.

**mumbled:** Imprecise pronunciation.

**musculoskeletal system:** Pertains to parts supporting and moving parts of the body, including the skeleton, tendons, and muscles.

**negativism:** Opposition to the suggestions of the interviewer to behave in a certain fashion.

**neglected:** Dress and personal hygiene indicate that the client is either incapable of or has disregarded their self-care.

**nervous system:** Pertains to collecting and processing information; it includes the brain, nerves, and neurotransmitters.

**obsessions:** Thoughts, feelings, or ideas that intrude upon a person's conscious awareness, and are accompanied by an effort to resist this intrusion and by an awareness that these thoughts are abnormal.

**olfactory hallucination:** A smell that does not have a concrete external stimulus.

**orientation:** The ability to identify oneself with respect to one's position in time, place, and person.

**overactive:** Excessive motor activity.

**overbearing:** Evincing a superior attitude, domineering, arrogant, proud, regarding others with disdain and as inferior, monopolizing.

**pacing:** Restlessness characterized by continual walking.

**panic:** An acute, intensive attack of anxiety associated with personality disorganization.

**paramnesia:** Disturbance of memory in which reality and fantasy are confused.

**perception:** The reception of many physical stimuli that bombard a person (sights, sounds, feelings, odours, tastes, and so on) and the mental processes where data is organized. Through perception, a person makes sense out of the many stimuli that bombard them.

**perplexity:** A pervasive feeling of bewilderment and uncertainty.

**persecutory delusions:** Over-suspiciousness leading to false persecutory ideas or beliefs.

**perseveration:** Pathological repetition of the same response to different questions.

**phobias:** An irrational fear of an object or situation and usually accompanied by behaviour to avoid that object or situation. In a phobia, the client retains the knowledge that their fear is unrealistic.

**plan:** A decision regarding method that would be used to harm oneself or another.

**pleasant:** Agreeable or harmonious.

**posture:** The position in which someone holds their body.

**poverty (paucity) of ideas:** Absence or scarcity of thoughts or imagination.

**preoccupation:** A state of daydreaming; the client appears to be out of touch with their surroundings and absorbed in their own thoughts.

**pressured:** Quality of speech; drivenness of the speech.

**proprioceptive hallucination:** A sensation of body posture without a concrete external stimulus. For example, a sensation that you are floating, when you are actually lying in your bed.

**quality:** Verbal and non-verbal fluctuations in tone.

**rambling:** A tendency to drift or wander from a subject.

**range:** The variation in emotional expression observed throughout the interview. It is characterized as full (normal variation in emotional expression) or constricted (limited variation in emotional expression).

**rate:** The speed of speech, which is further characterized as pressured (very rapid and difficult to interrupt), slowed, or appropriate.

**reactivity:** Whether or not one's mood changes in response to external events or circumstances.

**regressive:** Going back to a more infantile or immature level.

**relevant:** Related to the topic.

**repetitive:** Repetition of words or phrases.

**reproductive system:** Pertains to creating another; it includes sexual functioning.

**respiratory system:** Pertains to moving air in and out of the body; it includes the lungs.

**responsive:** Does not initiate conversation but will respond on approach.

**restless:** Unsettled, fidgety, wandering, agitated.

**retarded:** Movements are slow, laboured, and limited.

**rigid:** Gait and other movements appear stiff and puppet-like, which is indicative of severe lack of flexibility.

**sad:** Appears melancholic, depressed; reflecting misery, grief, and unhappiness.

**self-abusive:** Self-inflicted punishment and injury and acts of violence against one's self.

**self-centred:** Primarily concerned with one's own desires and needs, and indifferent to those of others.

**slowed:** Enunciation of words is prolonged or pauses between words are increased.

**somatic hallucination:** A physical experience that something is happening within the body without a concrete external stimulus.

**stability:** The consistency of mood, particularly within the course of a day.

**startle reaction:** Reflex motor response to a sudden, intense stimulus associated with a sudden increase in the level of consciousness. This can occur in anyone in an acute anxiety state.

**stereotypy:** A repetition of the motor action as is seen in chronic schizophrenic states. At times, it is highly organized and appears to be a ritualistic act.

**stuperose:** Lethargy in which the client is immobile, out of touch with their surroundings, and exhibits little or no response to stimuli.

**suicidal:** Intent to kill oneself.

**suspicious:** Distrustful and accusatory.

**tactile hallucination:** A feeling that does not have a concrete external stimulus.

**tangential thinking:** A disturbance in thinking in which the client is unable to express their ideas because they digress or are derailed in their thinking; they never quite get to the point.

**tantrums:** Uncontrolled, angry outbursts of bad temper.

**tearfulness:** Weepiness; moved to tears.

**thought flow:** The organization or "connectedness" of thinking. It is characterized as logical when there are clear and easily understood connections between thoughts, and as disjointed when these connections are unclear and difficult to follow.

**thought form:** The way (form) in which thoughts are expressed. It is characterized as concrete (inability to think beyond the most overt meaning), impoverished (little meaningful information contained in the conversation), or overly inclusive (excessive, irrelevant detail).

**thought rate:** May be revealed through direct questioning or inferred based on the rate of speech. It is characterized as rapid, slowed, or appropriate.

**tic:** Involuntary, spasmodic, repetitive motor movements of a small segment of the body.

**tremulous:** Movements that indicate impaired motor coordination, ranging from fine muscular tremors to spontaneous, spasmodic jerking.

**uncommunicative:** Unwilling or unable to verbalize.

**unkempt:** Dishevelled, inattentive to personal appearance or hygiene.

**visual hallucination:** Seeing something that does not have a concrete external stimulus.

**volition:** The ability of a person to make a choice and act on it.

**volume:** Power of sound; it is especially important to comment on if the volume of speech is unusually loud or hushed.

**whining:** Speech and tone are fretful, self-pitying, and complaintive.

**whispered:** Soft, breathy voice.

**willpower:** The determination to achieve.

**withdrawing:** Moving away from or retreating.

www.ingramcontent.com/pod-product-compliance
Lightning Source LLC
Chambersburg PA
CBHW081436270326
41932CB00019B/3219

* 9 7 8 1 7 7 3 3 8 0 7 0 4 *